I0441848

Never Knew I Wanted to be a Breast Cancer Survivor

Rebecca J Hogue

Published by Rebecca J Hogue, 2024.

NEVER KNEW I WANTED TO BE A BREAST CANCER SURVIVOR

First edition. February 18, 2024.

Copyright © 2024 Rebecca J Hogue.

ISBN: 978-0991854554

Written by Rebecca J Hogue.

Table of Contents

To my husband, Scott Drennan, who was my rock throughout this journey and continues to be my rock today!

Introduction

Being diagnosed with breast cancer at the age of 43, I was suddenly thrust into the world of the cancer patient. Having recently moved to California from Canada, I also had to deal with learning the ins and outs of a totally different healthcare system. As a blogger, I chose to use a blog to find meaning in my experiences, share my experiences, and to educate friends and loved ones about what it meant to really experience breast cancer as a 'young survivor' in a foreign and unfamiliar healthcare system.

I hope that my story helps other breast cancer patients and survivors feel a little less alone in the process. I hope that it helps friends and family better understand what their loved ones are going through. I hope it helps healthcare providers gain a deeper empathy for breast cancer patients.

It all started...

———

I t all started with denial. I felt something. Could it be what I was feeling was just a muscle strain? Surely if I waited a couple of days, it would go away.

I never thought I'd have to deal with breast cancer. When one of my relatives was diagnosed with breast cancer, she was the same age as me – 43. She had other risk factors and could trace breast cancer to the other side of her family, the side I wasn't related to. She died a year and a half after her diagnosis.

This should not be happening to me!

I was told that most women who get breast cancer do not have a family cancer history. As I wait for news from my doctor, I wonder: how is it possible that so many women get diagnosed with breast cancer without a family cancer history? Also, if the lifetime risk for getting breast cancer is one in eight, then how do those numbers add up?

I approach this new life challenge by using academic curiosity. I want to research and read the literature to figure out what I'm dealing with. Writing throughout the process lets me reflect and focus while giving me perspective. I decide to blog because it lets me journal my lived breast cancer experience and offer insights into the often-confusing medical jargon. I am starting to negotiate how this new identity changes who I am as an open academic.

Today my goal in life changes. *I want to be identified as a breast cancer survivor.* The alternative doesn't look so grand!

What should I hope for?

June 14, 2014

While I await the biopsy and other test results, I find myself uncertain and wondering – what should I be hoping for? If you are going to have breast cancer, the next question is, what kind of breast cancer? My problem is that I don't want to do a lot of reading about the different types of breast cancer right now. Instead, I only want to know about the best type to have, whatever that is, so I can hope that is what I have. But I don't know enough about breast cancer to have any idea of what I should be hoping for.

Anytime I feel the slightest bit of anything on the outer edges of my breast, I get concerned. Am I feeling cancer spread to my lymph nodes? I keep hoping that the cancer is localized and hasn't spread. Everything that I know about cancer tells me that spread would be considered bad news. Nothing is confirmed until the biopsy results come back, yet three different specialists weigh in by telling me that they would be "surprised if it isn't breast cancer."

Tears stream from my eyes as I focus on the current medical conditions tab in my online patient portal, where I see the words "breast cancer" for the first time. My hopes that it might not be breast cancer are shattered. Seeing it in writing for the first time is like a wave hitting me in the face and knocking me off my feet. Reality is starting to set in.

Now I ask myself, what should I be hoping for?

How do you prepare to lose a body part?

———

June 15, 2014

When the surgeon tells me that it is highly likely that I need a mastectomy, I do not internalize what that means. A new friend helps me understand the surgery's scope when she says that a mastectomy is like an amputation.

It becomes even more real when I realize my amputation-mastectomy could happen in the next two to three weeks. By July, I will likely not have my left breast.

I'm told that I need to think about reconstruction options. The "good news" is insurance companies are legally mandated to cover a patient's reconstructive surgery after breast cancer surgery. I must decide before my mastectomy because it will affect how the mastectomy surgery is done.

At first, I do not want a mastectomy if it means I will be lopsided and have just one breast. When I find out that there might be another malignant tumour in my right breast, and that I might end up with bilateral surgery, being unbalanced may not be an issue. One thing that plays into my decision is that I hate bras and wearing a prosthetic to make me look 'even' doesn't at all sound appealing.

I can logically think about what I want, and how this might play out, but I cannot emotionally prepare. I have no idea where to begin with the emotional side of this decision. How does one prepare to lose a body part?

Window shopping[1]

―――

June 16, 2014

My husband Scott and I often laugh at things that are absurd, but real, nonetheless. I recognize it clearly as a necessary coping mechanism but I know how easily something funny can turn into something sad.

When I was an undergraduate, one of my friends had a cancer recurrence. At her wedding shower, while she was sitting with the news that her cancer had come back, we were laughing about ridiculous wedding shower presents and cringe-worthy shower games—and then the focus of the jokes turned to wigs. There was laughing at first, followed by a sudden transition to tears. I remember her wedding shower turn of events every time I laugh about something. At any moment, that laugh can become a cry.

Today's laugh is about prosthetic breasts. I learn that there are special prosthetic breasts for swimming—aquadynamic breasts! They even make aerodynamic prosthetic breasts. Who knew? I was reminded of Aimee Mullins TED talk, "It's not fair having 12 pairs of legs." Aimee talks about how having various prosthetic legs allows her to be different heights. She talks about legs as things that allow her to have superpowers. For example, when she wants to run fast, she has special legs for that.

I laugh as my mind races—if I don't opt for reconstruction from my breast cancer surgery, then I, too, can have multiple sets of prosthetics for multiple purposes! I could have bigger breasts to fill out my favourite shirt, or smaller ones when I want to appear less noticeable. Then it occurs to me that people who see me regularly would find it rather odd if my chest size keeps changing. How would I go clothes shopping? Which breasts would I wear? If I were to get into competitive swimming, would the breasts I choose affect how fast I swim? Would that be considered cheating?

Wading into the morass of breast cancer surgical decision-making, means exploring my options. Reconstruction requires more complicated surgery and healing time. No reconstruction means a life of prosthetics.

As Scott and I walk around Sausalito, I notice other women's breasts. I never really noticed other women's breasts before, but now I am drawn to them and keep looking. I'm not even sure what I'm thinking when I'm looking. I laugh, then swallow tears. Prosthetics or not, I am window shopping.

[1] The story "Window Shopping" was published in Hogue (2016) *Agony and absurdity: Adventures in Cancerland.* Calcari Campbell, Hessen Pomeranz, & Bruns Worona (eds).

The speed of things

June 16, 2014

Everything is either too fast or too slow. I feel like the cancer is growing too fast. With each new ache in my body, I worry: Is this another symptom? Has it spread and reached my lymph nodes?

And things are too slow. I cannot even book appointments without the confirmation of an official pathology report. The good news is, the doctor and surgeon guarantee that they will fit me in when my pathology report comes back, which makes sense. They cannot recommend anything without all the report's vital information. Yet I want an appointment so that I know that I will not be waiting unnecessarily.

As the hours turn into days, I wonder if I am overreacting. What if it is just a 'minor' cancer? Since one in eight women will get breast cancer in their lifetime, is it that a big deal? A new friend points out a New York Times article (January 5, 2014), *Why Everyone Seems to have Cancer*, which she finds comforting. It argues that cancer is a 'normal' part of aging. Unfortunately, this doesn't help me at all. In some ways, it scares me, because I'm too young. Two-thirds of women with breast cancer are over 50. I'm not.

My life is on hold until I get clear data and information on my cancer. During this waiting period, the cancer is likely growing. But it does give me time to consider my options, exercise and get stronger, and think about how I want to spend my time over the next year. It is freeing to let go of things that I don't want to do.

I'm starting to get a new appreciation for sunk costs, which are .... When we make quality decisions, they should be based on the future, not the past. However, we tend to say, "But I've spent x years on this. I might as well finish it." Those x years represent a sunk cost from the past. Being told I have cancer helps me see the sunk costs of time, resources, and money affecting my decision-making. In the past, I've used long bike rides to clear my head. I know it is something that helps me both mentally and physically. Time for a nice long bike ride.

Impostor syndrome

June 16, 2014

I have a long conversation with my husband about chemotherapy. I am going through the mental preparations for when I will lose my hair. I have prepared myself mentally for the exploration of hair loss to the extent that I feel like I would be let down if that wasn't to be part of my journey.

Without that all-important confirmed pathology, I feel like a faker—as if I don't have breast cancer. What happens if I don't have cancer? Frankly, the large lump in my breast is convincing. What if it is just a minor cancer, have I been overreacting? Am I an impostor?

I miss a critical phone call when I am in the shower. The surgeon's voicemail says that my results are in. As I dial, the surgeon's words echo through my mind:

"Invasive Ductal Carcinoma (IDC) in both breasts... grade 3 in the left breast and grade 2 in the right breast. We will know more when the full report comes back."

I'm surprised to hear this information over the telephone but am also grateful to get this new medical update so quickly after the surgeon's outreach call. Learning about my cancer in small chunks gives me time to look things up and process the information before the next bit of news comes in.

A tough day

June 17, 2014

When I don't sleep well, I sure feel it the next day. Reality and fear are settling in. Does the blister on my hand mean anything? With every pain in my body, I wonder if the cancer has spread. An awareness of a new feeling in my breast is especially concerning. I wonder if the tumour is now reaching the chest wall. But the logical part of my brain says it could just be the biopsy healing – after all they did stick rather large needles in to extract core samples.

Telling people is hard – because it leads to reactions, questions, and conversations. I have learned to not tell anyone the news at the end of the night since it inevitably disrupts my sleep. The late day news of the second biopsy result is just as much to blame, I'm sure. I now point people to my blog, so that I don't have to keep repeating the same information. With each conversation, there is an emotional toll on both sides. Some people reach out and want to talk, but I'm not there yet. I cannot talk about it until I have enough information and a treatment plan.

I cannot plan or schedule anything without a treatment plan. I have no clue how sick I will be. I find myself thinking, "I need to do this before I get sick." My mind is telling me that the treatment is what will make me sick rather than the disease. When I got this diagnosis, I was in the midst of collecting data for my PhD. For the future, I'm wondering how much I should prepare so that I can pick up where I left off? Should I set up something that just keeps going while I'm away? And what do I just let go?

The role of fate in my life

June 17, 2014

Although I don't believe in a god per se, I do believe in fate. Throughout our bicycle journey (http://goingeast.ca/blog), my husband and I often felt that there was a higher being looking out for us.

Fate plays a role in helping me prepare for the challenges that lie ahead. In my professional life, fate directed me towards a PhD program, where I ended up working with the Department of Family Medicine (DFM). Without this, I never would have pursued work in medical education. Those last three years working with DFM meant I developed a much deeper understanding for how medical education works, how some aspects of medical research work (e.g. I know what implementation research is), and how medicine is practiced in an academic setting (even the difference between a community and academic setting). It's all very valuable knowledge as I learn to navigate the American health care system. Developing friendships with so many physicians from my work with DFM strengthens my support system.

The PhD program helped me discover myself as a blogger. It helped me create an overlapping wide-reaching social network – which I am very grateful for. When I first heard that I had cancer, I had people that I reach out to. These friends put me in touch with other friends – all helping to form a network of support. In times of crisis, we discover the true power of being part of networked communities.

And so, it begins

June 18, 2014

We receive some mixed news about the pathology: the cancer in both breasts is IDC (invasive ductal carcinoma). Both are also ER-positive and PR-positive, called hormone positive. We don't know yet about HER2 because that test takes longer. Hormone positive is a good thing, as it means there are more drug treatment options. The nurse navigator phoned me after first following up with the surgeon. She collected and shared with me all the info I needed. Her awesome work saves me an immense amount of time, which is very useful.

Today we will find out what all this means in meetings with the surgeon and medical oncologist at the local clinic. Tomorrow, we will get a second opinion at Stanford.

I'm torn between the two environments since my choice determines what the treatment options are and who is best suited to doing them. The local clinic has provided excellent service so far. It is easy to get in to see people and I have access to my care providers via email with one catch: apparently, the system will not let them email malignant pathology, so I request printed copies of my reports.

I'm not interested in nipple sparing surgeries and things that are done to help with cosmetic reconstruction at the university hospital. Honestly, I cannot see putting myself through unnecessary surgeries to save skin that might be diseased. More on that later.

Priorities

———

June 18, 2014

Time is my biggest challenge right now. Things are moving so very quickly as I manage many different appointments, phone calls, blog posts, notifications, and minutiae.

My number one priority pre-surgery is biking. Back when I thought I might have cancer (after my family doc appointment), I decided I would train so that I could be strong and in the best physical shape possible before surgery and chemo. This means allocating two to three hours a day or more for biking.

My second priority is to have some fun. Years ago, I read the book *From chocolate to morphine: Everything you need to know about mind-altering drugs* (Rosen & Weil, 2004), which talked about finding things that cause your natural high – like when you were a kid and you would spin around really fast. One of the things that causes that natural high for me is sailing. So, we are looking for ways to go sailing regularly. However, sailing can be very physically demanding, which will likely be a challenge. This Saturday, we are headed up to San Francisco to sail on a 2003 America's Cup boat. If we enjoy it, and there are less strenuous ways to participate, we may consider buying a season crew membership, which would allow us to go sailing most weekends. This means we could spend every Saturday or Sunday going out for a sail for as long as my body allows. Here is hoping that we enjoy it!

Double-mastectomy and chemo

―――――

June 19, 2014

If I'm repeating myself, I apologize. Over the last two or three days, my short-term memory sucks. I cannot seem to hold thoughts for that long. I very often walk into a room having completely forgotten why I was there. Worse is that I sit in front of the computer intent on doing something, then have no clue what that was. It feels like I am easily drawn in many different directions.

Today we met the surgeon and then oncologist at the local clinic. I also missed a call from the social worker.

There isn't exactly a plan for treatment yet, just some general recommendations based upon the known pathology. There is a key test called the HER2 which should be ready early next week. The preliminary HER2 was inconclusive, so they send samples to a different lab for further testing. To simplify the discussion with the oncologist, we only go over options that make sense for HER2 negative, which is 80% likely.

I have two separate cancers, one in each breast. The surgeon's recommendation is a double-mastectomy. I had come to the same conclusion when the biopsy results for the right breast came back positive. What is interesting here is that prior to having cancer, I always thought that if this happened to me, I'd want it out immediately. Now that I have cancer, I'm not as certain; yes, I want it out, but the decision over chemo or surgery first leads to more thinking.

I decide I will not do reconstruction, which makes the surgery much simpler. The mastectomy involves removing all breast tissue, including the nipples. Reconstruction brings a lot of risks, and frankly, I'd be happy to never need to wear a bra again! I've never really liked the way my nipples looked. I've not had kids, so I don't have that connection to them either. With reconstruction, I'd likely lose all or most feeling, so if they are not a source of sexual pleasure, then there isn't a lot of point to keeping them, especially when nipple sparing surgery is both more complex and can potentially increase the chance of recurrence. Choosing to not do the nipple sparing surgery for those reasons is logical. I like logical. It is a relief to make this big decision that will change my body forever.

Both cancers (left and right) have the same characteristics (HR-positive and PR-positive). Given the growth rate of the left, chemotherapy is recommended. The chemo would be the ACT type (assuming HER2 negative). Don't know too much about the chemo yet, since we just learned about the recommendation today. The chemo could happen before or after surgery, so this is the big question right now.

Now if I am HER2 positive, that means that chemo will happen first, since there are some chemotherapies that can block the HER2 protein that can only be given before surgery. There are complexities with HER2 – including an increase mortality rate. If you are inclined to pray, pray for HER2 negative on both sides.

I've learned that statistics only mean something before you get a diagnosis. They provide hope (e.g. 80% of breast cancers are HER2 negative), but they mean nothing once you receive the diagnosis. It is no longer relevant what the statistics are, like 1 in 8 women will get breast cancer in their lifetime or that a certain percentage of breast cancers are HR and PR positive. Both cancers are positive. Statistics only matter for the unknown future, not the known present.

Having two cancers is not so common, but it certainly makes the double-mastectomy question easier. If I only had one cancer, keeping the second breast would have been expected unless I have one of the breast cancer genes, such as BRCA. But that information won't be available for a couple of weeks. We are hoping for negative here too. I would have then had a harder decision regarding reconstruction. Having only one cancerous breast would have always had me wondering if keeping the right breast would mean an increased risk of recurrence, and it would mean mammograms every six months on the right breast, and constant worry. Plus, it would have been harder to figure out clothing and all those complexities. Yes, women do it, but I would have found it difficult – a constant reminder. The double-mastectomy is one of the easier decisions.

Tomorrow, we go for a second opinion at Stanford. It is also a chance to see Stanford and decide if it is a better treatment option. The folks at the local clinic saw no reason I would get any different treatment at Stanford given what we know now. The only thing that might matter is if there is a clinical trial that I qualify for at Stanford that isn't available at the local clinic. The local clinic oncologist didn't know of any. Stanford in some ways has the coolness and prestige factor – I could say I went there, and I'd wear the sweatshirt with pride. But it is also at least another 20 minutes further away, and parking costs $12. Parking is free at the local clinic and most of the locations are within a 5 to 15-minute drive from my husband's office and a 20-minute drive from home. This all adds up.

So far, the care at the local clinic has been superb. Although I might have been leaning towards Stanford late last week, I'm now leaning the other direction. But tomorrow will tell. I may get to Stanford and feel that everything is right there. I am happy to know that I have choices. Choice means that I have some sense of control and I'm a control freak. With most of this, I don't have any control. I'll take what I can get!

A long day

———

June 19, 2014

Our day begins with an early drive to Stanford so that we avoid rush-hour traffic. We enter the main floor of the cancer centre, searching for breakfast and a good cup of coffee, where we walk past an older lady in a wheelchair, bald and with bags under her eyes. There is a man nearby wearing a mask that reminds me of the gas masks in movies. I feel the sickness here.

The breakfast options suck, but at least the coffee is good.

We have a consult with the breast surgeon, and they booked a breast MRI. I'll only do the MRI here if I decide to get treatment here, as each surgeon likes to have the MRI from a specific machine.

"Please undress from the waist up and put the gown on with the ties in the front," instructs the medical assistant as she closes the curtain and leaves the room. I change and feel the chill. I must remember to bring a sweater next time.

The surgeon enters the room. She is petite and about 10 years older than me. I sense her confidence. We immediately feel the difference between her, a female surgeon who specializes in breast cancer surgery, as compared to the general surgeon at the local clinic who did the initial biopsy.

After a quick exam, she gets straight to the point. "From a surgery standpoint you have a couple of options. You can have a double mastectomy, or you can have lumpectomies, which would result in two smaller breasts. I'd like you to consult with a plastic surgeon before you make your decision."

The idea of a plastic surgeon is foreign to me. I remember a friend commenting that she thought I was moving to "silicone valley" rather than "Silicon Valley", referring to the cosmetic surgeries that are common in Hollywood. At the mention of a plastic surgeon, the vision of breast enhancing cosmetic surgery floats through my mind.

"Research shows that the 10–15-year recurrence rates are the same for double mastectomy and lumpectomy plus radiation. This is your decision," she emphasizes, "I want you to think about what will make you happy in the longer term. My goal is to have the best outcome. This is not just about removing the cancer, rather it is your longer-term happiness." It is clear to me that she has a passion for what she does. I feel like I can trust her.

"I would like you to see one of my colleagues, a medical oncologist. I have a colleague here that can see you now." She leaves the room. My husband and I look at each other. I'm sure that he can see the fear in my eyes.

A man about 10 years older than me walks into the room and introduces himself. I immediately like him. He asks to examine me, then walks to the sink to wash his hands. He examines me first sitting up and then laying down. He makes note of the lump that he feels in the left breast, measuring the size and distance from the nipple. The lump in the right breast is a little trickier. He isn't sure if he is feeling the lump or the wound from the biopsy. He checks my armpits, feeling for enlarged lymph nodes. Fortunately, he doesn't feel any.

"Looking at your initial biopsy results and the initial scans, neo-adjuvant chemotherapy may be a good option". He explains that neo-adjuvant means chemotherapy before surgery. "We need to wait for the results of the HER2 test before we can determine the type of chemotherapy, but first we need to see the results of the MRI". He then leaves the room.

My husband and I are watching the clock. I have a 4pm appointment for the MRI, and we are quickly running out of time.

The oncologist returns with the surgeon. They both agree that they need the MRI results as well as the HER2 results before recommending a specific treatment plan. They emphasize that I have options, and I will need to make some choices, but right now we are running out of time. I am told to book follow up appointments for Monday and go get the MRI.

"Lie down on the bed, chest down with your breasts in the holes, hands above your head" the MRI technician says to me, with a caring inflection in his voice.

I follow the directions of the MRI tech. I can feel the IV in my arm tug a little as I hop onto the cold bed and position myself. Lying on my stomach with my breasts sticking down through the holes, I think about how surreal this entire experience is. The MRI tech places earmuffs on my head and asks, "Are you comfortable?" I wouldn't exactly call this position comfortable, but I can manage it.

"I'll be just on the other side of the glass. Squeeze the ball if you need out of the machine. I will talk to you throughout the scan. OK?" he asks as he prepares to leave the room and begin collecting the images that will help determine the extent of my cancer.

I feel my elbows bumping up against the sides as the bed slowly moves into the MRI machine. I am surprised by just how small it is. I'm thankful that I'm looking down and not up, so that I don't feel that my world is collapsing in on me. I take a deep breath.

"The first scan will be two minutes", I hear him say through the MRI speakers. Then it begins. A whirring that reminds me of passing fire trucks, followed by clicking and shaking. Whirs, honks, and other sounds that remind me of the sounds of the alarms and shakes of the first container ship we travelled on back in 2008 when doing our around the world bicycle trip. I'm transported to the Bahamas, watching as the cranes that remind me of the four legged creatures in Star Wars load and stack containers, shaking the entire ship when the large deck covers are put in place. I am brought back to reality when the tech says, "We are going to put in the contrast now. You will feel a warm sensation. The next scan will be five minutes".

After forty-five minutes of scans, we are finished for the day. We take back roads to avoid rush hour traffic. Back at home, we both collapse. It has been a long day.

Throughout this process, everyone has been very clear to highlight that breast cancer treatment is an individual choice. They provide you with the options and, in the end, you need to be the one that decides which option to take. I feel like the treatment options being discussed at the local clinic are more traditional than those at Stanford. I get the sense that Stanford deals with people with more aggressive cancers, but also with rare cases. At the local clinic, I didn't see any sick people, so I didn't feel like I was sick. After seeing all the sickness at Stanford, for the first time, I feel like I too am sick.

A new friend gives me some great advice to help choose a healthcare team: "Choose who you want to trust, and then trust them". I feel that I can trust both this new surgeon and oncologist.

Caution – this one talks about death

Yesterday, after two hours of climbing, I successfully rode my bike to the top of Mount Hamilton from the fire station. That's seven miles up a hill that used to be a horse cart path and is now a paved road. Throughout the climb I found myself stopping in shaded corners to both catch my breath and cry. When I think about what is to come, I put on a brave face, but I still find myself crying.

I am struck by how some things are now clear. When we were creating our wills before we went on our Going East bike tour (http://goingeast.ca), I didn't think I liked the idea of my body being used for research. Now, I definitely my body to be used for research or medical education. I think my time working with doctors and doing research has changed my opinion on this. I also have clarity as to where I'd like my ashes spread – over the molten lava on Hawaii's big island. These are things that I couldn't figure out before, but now just seem to make sense. They don't feel like big decisions even though they are.

Also, I don't want to know my prognosis, which is a statistical measurement of your likelihood to survive. The only measure that matters to me is me, and no statistic can tell me that. But the prognosis statistic is a helpful measure to determine treatment options. Those are the statistics I want to know.

I rush to find my phone and answer it just in time. The surgeon from the local clinic gets straight to the point: "The tumour board met and reviewed your biopsy results. Regardless of the HER2 status, we recommend that you do chemotherapy before surgery. Chemotherapy can start within the next two weeks. First you will need to get a mediport. I can do that and at the same time do a sentinel node biopsy which will tell us if the cancer has spread to your lymph nodes. We cannot yet recommend a specific chemotherapy as that would depend on the HER2 status. We also need to wait for insurance approval which can take a week."

It feels good to at least have a recommendation; however, I am still leaning towards treatment at Stanford. As a Canadian, I find the idea of needing to wait for insurance approval before getting treatment dumbfounding. Why should insurance determine treatment options?

Support group

———

June 22, 2014

After sailing this morning, my husband strongly encourages me as he drops me off at a newly-diagnosed-and-in-treatment breast cancer support group. I am hesitant and rather nervous because I haven't told anybody in person that I have cancer. It isn't easy saying it out loud.

"Hi, I'm Becky", I say as tears start streaming down my face. In a quivering voice, I say "Last Thursday I was told I have bilateral breast cancer, IDC in both breasts..."

The support group makes it easier to talk about because it gives me a safe space to say it out loud, but also a place to talk about it in shared and understood cancer language. Too bad there isn't a PhD student breast cancer support group, where people understand my academic speak. I also meet a couple of nice people. Since we know so few people in California, it seems odd to me, but the cancer support groups are likely where we will develop new friendships. I am encouraged to come back to both that group and the young survivor group and want to give it a try. We hope they restart the couples' group – as 'Scott and Becky' could use a support group too, not just Becky.

Why me? ... it is what it is.

―――

June 23, 2014

I hear others say things like, 'Why me?' and I'm somewhat surprised that I have yet to have that feeling. Perhaps it is a bit of denial? Is it related to my outlook on life? I'm not a theist, that is I don't believe in a god. I remember lying in bed chatting with my husband about the possibility of cancer before the diagnosis. We said, 'It is what it is – we will deal with it.' There has yet to be the 'why me' feeling. Perhaps by not believing in a god, it means that I don't have anyone to ask that question to?

I see the world as some form of random chance. I do believe some things happen for a reason. My past experiences working with the Department of Family Medicine in Ottawa has helps me understand the medical world that I'm now immersed in.

I'm not anti-spiritual and find peace communing in nature. Today we walked for 9km at Big Basin Redwoods State Park, which is a record distance for me. The trees are 1000s of years old and it's one of my favourite places. There is a special energy when I am walking and touching these ancient trees – some with battle scars from fires long past. They are survivors.

We sat for an hour on a bridge over a dribbling creek and noticed these water bugs that create the most fascinating shadows on the bottom – like moving black dots. It is amazing and fascinating what you see when you slow down for a few minutes and just be.

Today was a good day.

Why I take selfies

———

June 23, 2014

When we first explored treatment at Stanford, it occurred to me that I wanted a series of pictures of me, taken at the same place, every time we go. I wanted a nice tree behind me. There are a bunch of giant Eucalyptus trees, which seem to be constantly shedding their bark. There is something symbolic in that, as the trees shed their bark, I shall be shedding my hair. When all this is over, I shall have a time lapsed video that shows a series of pictures of me as I progress through this process - both evidence and testimonial to my journey.

Right now, I'm having Scott take lots of pictures of me. If I don't make it, I want there to be lots of happy pictures of me and for family and friends to see that I am doing well right now. I am strong and want to show it through pictures. I may need these pictures when I'm going through treatment, to remind myself where I was before this began, and where I want to come back to.

Knowing what to expect

June 24, 2014

In my experience, fear comes from not knowing what to expect and not feeling you have any control over what's about to happen. When you feel helpless, you're far more afraid than you would be if you knew the facts. If you're not sure what to be alarmed about, everything is alarming. (Hadfield, 2013)

Today we got a couple of interesting lab results back. First, the HER2 FISH test came back negative. This is good, as the HER2 treatments aren't great on your heart and last longer. What it means is that the type of cancer I have is the type that is most common, and most understood.

The MRI also showed something interesting. Rather than having a large 4cm+ tumour in my left breast, I have two smaller tumours (2cm and 3cm). I'm not completely certain how to take this information, as I now have three tumours. However, the treatment for one is the same as the treatment for the other – so from a treatment perspective nothing changes – and I don't have a 'big' tumour. The MRI also showed no indication of node involvement – which means I caught it early.

Decisions come in pairs. The first choice is chemo first or surgery first. The next choice depends on the first, but either way, when it comes to surgery, I will need to decide on whether I want a mastectomy or a lumpectomy plus radiation. Whatever I do on one side, I'll do on the other – symmetry matters to me. The medical statistical data tells me what choices I have, that is, it narrows things down, but I need to make the decision using my gut.

After confirming that chemo was advised regardless of surgery choice (increased prognosis by 10% in cases like mine), and that chemo before or after surgery didn't make a difference in the prognosis, but could make surgery easier, the first decision I made was to go with chemo first. My gut had been telling me this for quite some time. I just feel like this cancer came out of nowhere and is spreading, and the only way to catch it systemically is with chemo.

Of course, that wasn't the only decision – because every decision leads to another decision. Now I need to choose between two chemo regimes. The quantitative numbers say they have the same outcomes based on clinical trials.

The two options look something like this:

Option 1: doxorubicin and cyclophosphamide (AC) followed by paclitaxel (T) in the form of 1 treatment every 2 weeks of AC for 4 cycles, followed by one treatment per week of T for 12 cycles.

Option 2: docetaxel (T) and cyclophosphamide (C) in the form of 1 treatment every 3 weeks of TC for 6 cycles.

They are given at different intervals, but I've decided that the logistics of intervals is not an important variable for me. Some people chose one over the other based upon convenience of treatment and the latter option requires less visits and less infusions. I am going to choose based upon side effects, and which seem less likely to be problematic with my body.

After the doctors' appointments, we walk around the arboretum on the campus and find the perfect old eucalyptus tree for my picture series. The tree hasn't yet shed its bark for this season so it is showing older growth now; as the weeks pass the shedding will show the underlying new growth.

Significance of dates and getting ready for chemo

June 26, 2014

It is funny how special dates have meaning – and how we know what dates are good and which are not. I want to strongly avoid starting chemo on July 1st, as I did not want every Canada Day to be a reminder.

Instead, the date aligns with a date that already has meaning for me. July 7 is my father's birthday. On July 7, 2008, Scott and I left our house and hopped on our bikes to begin a 16-month trip around the world (http://goingeast.ca/blog/2008/07/07/we-left-home-finally/).

On July 7, 2014, I start chemo and will also start writing the going east book. I had done a little writing for National Novel Writing Month (NaNoWriMo) the year before I started my PhD but haven't picked it up since. When I thought I might have cancer, the only real regret I had in life was that I had not yet written the Going East book. My chemo start date is the opportunity to start writing the book. I'll bring my laptop with me to treatment and see if I can use at least some of that time for writing.

We went to chemo class today, which confirmed a lot of what we already knew. We were able to reduce our worries about some of the excessive precautions listed in the "Understanding Chemotherapy: A guide for patients and families" by the American Cancer Society. It provided some horribly scary recommendations – saying things like for the first 48-hours we need to be careful not to exchange bodily fluids, and we shouldn't use the same toilet, and that whoever cleans should wear two pairs of rubber gloves. Scott is looking up the sources in the academic literature to see if there is any merit. When I mention this to one of the many nurses I talk to, she thought I was crazy and recommended the website http://chemocare.com/ for chemo care information.

Tomorrow I will have my port put in. They use what is called twilight sedation, which means I will be awake but not completely aware of everything. In theory, the port scar will heal within a couple of days. I am hoping that I can hop in the pool within a week, as I suspect that swimming may be one of my better post-chemo options because it's easier on the joints.

I've also asked three friends to be my exercise accountability buddies throughout chemo. I could use one or two more volunteers. In the PhD process some people use writing accountability buddies to help them stay motivated to get through writing their proposal or dissertation. An exercise accountability buddy is someone to hassle me to get off the couch on those days when I just don't feel like it. I don't want to overdo exercise, but they recommend trying to keep to the same level of exercise throughout chemo, but with more rest time. Since I mostly bike 1.5-3 hours per day (4-5 times per week), that might be a bit too much to maintain all the time. It would be nice if I could at least make sure I'm doing something every day that isn't a chemo or procedure day.

I experienced anger for the first time today. When I was biking, I found myself angry that the treatment for breast cancer is to cut it off. How archaic is it that the treatment for disease is amputation? I'm expecting that either tomorrow with the installation of the port, or July 7th with the first chemo treatment, the whole 'I have cancer' thing will sink in and I'll start to realize what this all means. Right now, I'm just taking things one procedure at a time. I'm trying to make sure we have everything organized and in place for the time 'when I get sick', because I don't feel sick now.

TV breast cancer

―――

June 29, 2014

I don't watch a lot of TV, so my perceptions may be off, but I'm still a little mad. When someone on TV gets breast cancer, they don't portray it right at all in my opinion. They don't show you the decisions that need to be made, rather they seem to always show someone going through chemo – which many women with breast cancer don't do. They don't show surgery – which pretty much all women with breast cancer go through. By dramatizing the whole experience, they do nothing to prepare you for the reality of it. This really does makes me rather mad!

When one of the lead characters on Parenthood had breast cancer last year, she lost her hair, got sick, and ended up in the hospital because she ignored an infection. However, they never dealt with breast cancer's surgical implications, mainly: what it means to not have a breast after having a part of your body cut off. Yes, I am in a phase of expressing anger.

I'm also annoyed at our society. The entire concept of reconstruction is so much more emphasized here in the U.S., where it feels like the land of fake boobs. From what I understand, many people choose techniques that use their own body fat rather than silicone implants. People will think I am weird if I do not opt for reconstruction. I question all these non-essential surgeries and the extra pains that women go through. Why would I subject myself to that? Many of the women I know going through reconstruction did not have chemo – so they had one less toxic experience with breast cancer.

I'm feeling strong. With each passing day, the port wound is healing. I'm hoping for a longer bike ride today – and might try one of my upright bikes. I should be able to swim by next week, depending on when the third biopsy occurs. By not having surgery first, I'm losing some certainty in the cancer – as they cannot fully stage it until it is removed, and full pathology is done. The imaging doesn't provide enough detail. To go from one larger tumour to two smaller ones under MRI (which was not seen on ultrasound and mammogram) demonstrates how inaccurate imaging can be.

Questions remain: Is the tumour getting smaller on its own? Is it spontaneously curing itself?

I'm an educator

July 5, 2014

A couple weeks ago, I reflected on who I am. I am an academic, but further reflection has me now questioning what type of academic. Since diagnosis, I haven't been able to read a single academic article. I've browsed through a few, but my concentration and interest have not been there. I may not be approaching this 'cancer' problem as an academic, but I do want to approach it as an educator.

I don't call myself a teacher, which I define as a person who leads K-12 classrooms. I educate teachers and doctors on how to use technology.

As an instructional designer, I also educate through my writing. I create training programs and packages designed to help professionals learn new skills.

I wonder how my cancer can be turned into an educational experience. Who would I educate? How can I make the most out of this experience from an educational point of view?

First, I want people to learn what a breast lump feels like. I wish more residents were taking an interest and learning from my experience in my care at Stanford. I had no idea what a cancerous lump felt like, even when it happened to me. One memory that stands out is from my secondary school's health education class. The nurse brought in a mannequin breast, yet I could never find its lump. At home, inspecting my young teenaged breasts made me wonder if everything under the skin was a lump. I had pretty lumpy breasts but not a lot of fatty breast tissue back then.

I was never good at laying down in bed and checking once a month but did habitually inspect my breasts every time I showered. After my June 1st bike ride, there was a new firm area, which is how I knew that something had changed. I didn't realize that it was cancer. I thought that the somewhat rough bike ride on a dirt path caused a strain. My breast wasn't sore, it was just solid. In young women under forty-five, most breast cancers are found through self-examination – you feel something has changed. Being able to notice these changes is what matters.

It's a little-known fact that although you are at increased risk for breast cancer if an immediate family member has had it, "about 85% of breast cancers occur in women who have **no family history of breast cancer.** These occur due to genetic mutations that happen as a result of the aging process and life in general, rather than inherited mutations." (http://www.breastcancer.org/symptoms/understand_bc/statistics). Although there is a lot of press about the hereditary breast cancers, for most women, a diagnosis is completely unexpected. When women think no one in their family has had breast cancer, it hinders screening because they think it couldn't happen to them. Breast cancer was never a concern for me, although I still inspected my boobs every time I got in the shower, cause, why not?

So, all you women out there, get in the habit every time you jump in the shower, especially if you are too young for routine mammograms!

Joining the cancer blogosphere

────

July 6, 2014

I have been blogging for a few weeks now but remain hesitant to read other people's cancer blogs or reach out to others who are going through similar experiences due to fear and denial.

I am part of several online communities where I find friendship, strength, and much needed support. But, to join a cancer community means to admit that I have cancer. There is more to it than that – it is the fear of joining a community, developing solid friendships, and then losing people in that community. I'm OK with admitting I have cancer, but not OK admitting that it is something that might one day kill me. I don't want to deal with the death of a good friend – and so, I hesitate to reach out to others who are also going through this experience.

Yet I realize that I need to read and learn from others. There is also a pull to share my experiences, so that others can learn from me. My need drives me to participate in online communities and face-to-face support groups. I do it with hesitation and a bit of fear. I'm afraid to get too close to anyone who I might lose.

I'm ready

———

July 6, 2014

I am so ready to make the transition from someone with breast cancer to someone fighting breast cancer. Tomorrow morning, bright and early, I begin chemotherapy – assuming the heart ultrasound and blood tests say I'm healthy. I find the idea of being in 'excellent health' and having cancer at the same time rather ironic.

My 'cancer' bag that I bring with me when I go up to Stanford for the day is laid out. It's a handy gift from a local breast cancer support organization that hosts Saturday afternoon support group. I bought a new t-shirt with a low neckline so that my port is easily accessible.

My cancer bag includes:

- A nice warm blanket/wrap that I received from the church where my in-laws go (thank-you).
- A scarf that I received from my friend Maha in Egypt (thank-you).
- A teddy bear that Scott brought me when I was in the hospital for surgery before we were married (with the Canadian connection Hudson Bay sweater).

- Some snacks and electrolyte mixes to add to my water bottle.

- My cancer treatment binder, which includes a bunch of cards and the caring card I received from the Ottawa First Unitarian Congregation (thank-you), the card my mom sent with a hope rock on it, and various post cards sent from distant friends (thank-you).
- Headphones, so I can watch TV or listen to music or podcasts. I have a collection of preloaded Vinyl Cafe Stories and Under the Influence

podcasts.

I will also bring my laptop, iPad, and iPhone. I have no idea what I'm going to feel like doing during chemo. Scott will help lug my stuff – bringing both the laptop and iPad seems a little redundant, but if I am in the mood for any serious writing (beyond blogging), my laptop has Scrivener on it. Plus, my laptop lets me watch Canadian network TV shows, which I cannot do on my iPad.

I've learned that chemo side effects vary by the person. I'll either be tired or overly energetic for the first few days and then tired towards the end of the cycle. If you know me, you know that I like to plan things. This whole uncertainty over how I will react is driving me crazy. I just need to know if I'll be able to get some work done or not.

Since diagnosis, my life has been focused around improving my health. That means lots of long bike rides and long walks, enjoying sailing, and going to Yosemite; various medical tests, scans and appointments; and learning about my breast cancer treatment options. I put all my contract work on hold and am starting to go stir crazy. I hope to get back to some of that work – however, I just don't know how I will react to chemo, so I'm afraid to jump into anything right now. The waiting game continues ... today I wait ... I'm going to swim and go to the market. Now that my stomach is sorted, we need some food in the house – although chemo may change that too.

First day of chemo

—————

July 7, 2014

Step one is going to the infusion treatment area (ITA) to have my port accessed. I watch intently as the nurse opens the kit and cleans my skin around the port with an alcohol swab. Next, she places the special needle directly into the port. She draws blood and flushes the line with saline. I have the sensation of smell coming from the inside of my body as she slowly pushes saline into the IV to prevent blood from clotting in the IV.

Before the oncologist appointment, we walk over to my tree for photos, which captures my roiling emotions and trepidation. I also put on a brave face and forced smile for the second photo.

I then have a brief appointment with my oncologist where he validates that my blood tests indicate that I'm healthy enough for chemo.

We check in at the infusion treatment area (ITA) desk. Five minutes later, the nurse calls my name and directs me to a chair. I find the control and adjust the angle of the back rest and the height of the footrest. It is a little chilly, so I place my blanket over my lap, and find a crook in the chair for my teddy bear.

The nurse returns and connects my port to a saline drip that runs through the infusion monitor. She gives me a pill cup with pre-meds: a cocktail of anti-nausea drugs and steroids to both counteract the side effects and to make the chemo more effective. I feel a mix of sadness and fear at the sight of the medication.

We wait 30 minutes for the pre-meds to take effect. The nurse returns with the Doxorubicin, the A in the AC regime, also known as the red devil because of the colour and the possibility that it can damage your heart. The nurse checks the package from the pharmacy, asks me my name and birthdate. She shows me the label and asks me to validate that it correctly shows my name and birthdate.

She then calls over a second nurse, and they repeat the process, asking me my name and birthdate and validating my medical record number as well as the medication and dosage.

The nurse connects the first syringe to the IV bag. Tears well up in my eyes, as reality sets in. She quickly closes the curtain and begins to slowly push the Doxorubicin into my IV line which mixes with saline and then flows into my body through the port. She watches me closely to ensure that I'm not having an adverse reaction such as shortness of breath or heart palpitations. When the first vial empties after a couple of minutes, we move onto the second one. The nurses serenade the person in the chair across from me, "Hey now, your chemo is done". I look forward to hearing those words.

Once the Doxorubicin finishes, we again wait to ensure there are no adverse reactions. After 20 minutes, the nurse opens Cyclophosphamide (C), the next bag of chemotherapy, and we again go through the name and birthdate validation process. A second nurse comes over and validates that the medication is correct. She then hooks up the IV to mix with the saline at the rate specified on the infusion machine. I notice a weird metallic smell coming from inside my body. After an hour of watching TV, the IV bag is empty, and the infusion machine starts beeping.

After four hours, the first treatment is done. The nurse removes the IV from my port and sends me home with instructions on who to call if I experience any adverse reactions. Done for the day, or so we think.

So far, so good.

Pains with the American System

July 7, 2014

Having decent insurance makes most of the process of cancer treatment go smoothly. With a week of advanced notice, we thought it was all figured out ... but not so much.

The chemo went well today. I'm feeling a little stressed and just took something for that. I'm not sure if worrying about nausea is causing nausea or if I'm feeling nausea. We wait until the anti-anxiety meds kick in to decide if I need another anti-nausea pill. I have several options, so all is good.

I'm supposed to get a Neulasta shot tomorrow, used to boost the white blood cell count. The insurance company won't approve going to the university clinic for the shot – rather, I'm supposed to do it myself. My chemo nurse gave us a lesson on how to do a subcutaneous injection in between skin and fat, like an insulin injection. It is more convenient, since Scott can give it to me after work, rather than him having to take more time off work to drive up to the university clinic for a simple needle.

Getting the actual medication is a problem. The university clinic put the order into my pharmacy, but the insurance wouldn't go through. Neulasta shots are about $4000 each. The pharmacy called the university clinic who tried to get it approved, only to be told that we needed to make the request (i.e., it couldn't be made on behalf of us). We called, to be told that there is no pre-authorization, which means that the university clinic needs to call to do an urgent pre-authorization. Once we hear that the pre-authorization is done, Scott needs to call back our pharma care insurance provider, and have a supervisor do an override. Once we get the override, then our local pharmacy can fill the prescription. However, this all needs to happen before 8pm tonight as the pharmacy doesn't stock Neulasta. It is already after 4pm, therefore, they need to order it today so that it arrives by mid-day tomorrow.

If we don't get the insurance approval until tomorrow, we will need to find a pharmacy that stocks Neulasta, either Stanford or hopefully the local cancer clinic, as they are closer.

One way or another it will happen. It is just a lot more drama than I would have liked. Not sure why this pre-authorization requirement didn't surface sooner as they have known for over a week that I was starting chemo today. But, as the saying goes, 'It is what it is' ... we shall deal with it.

Negotiating identities in multiple worlds

July 8, 2014

I live between two worlds negotiating my different identities.

Anyone who gets breast cancer under 45 is a 'young survivor', so I'm renegotiating what it means to be a young cancer patient. In church, we had groups for young adults aged 18-35 and I remember the very awkward transition that happened as I could not relate to the younger group. We ended up starting our own group of 30-40 somethings to discuss spiritual and life issues that better aligned with where we were in life.

With the cancer groups, I relate to the 55ish year-old women who have established professional careers. I relate but don't have the same kind of cancer. When they hear of my cancer, it scares them, because is it not what the first nurse navigator called "old lady cancer". These survivors have slow growing cancers with positive outcomes in the range of 95-98%.

The young cancer survivors usually have more aggressive cancers and are often raising young children or early teens. Some have great support, but others amazingly power through cancer treatment without asking for help from their families. From this perspective, I'm not that strong. Perhaps I am a little wiser. My yearlong bike trip showed me that sometimes it is better for the people in your lives if you provide concrete ways to help.

My empathy for others has increased. Although I blog a lot about how I'm feeling, I worry about how others will feel when they read it. What will help others understand?

I forget to send out thank-you notes because I cannot keep track of it all. I greatly appreciate support and kind words. I hope my short thank-you here is enough for others to understand that they too are in my thoughts and heart.

I had to give myself permission to nap

July 9, 2014

I n all my pushes to make sure I'm getting enough exercise; I lost sight of my need for sleep. I got quite a bit of sleep last night, but by 2pm was knackered. I should stop pushing myself and just take a nap ... two hours later I woke up feeling refreshed.

The advice I get varies by who is giving it. Nurses tend to provide advice on the extreme side of things: absolutely no alcohol, swimming, or biking. They tend to provide advice based upon the worst-case scenario, but also discount mental health. Exercise is important to my mental health. The oncologist explains the chemo cycle and says it is OK to swim the first week, but as my white blood counts get low, I should stop swimming until the counts return. He said it was OK to have the occasional glass of wine, but don't get fall-down drunk because they are worried about low platelets leading to excessive bleeding. There is a period in the middle of a treatment cycle when infection is of greater concern. I don't need to be overly cautious all the time, especially at the cost of my mental health.

I'm not sure if the chemo smell is something that I'm experiencing from the inside or the outside. I'm not at the 48-hour mark yet, so I could still be excreting the chemo in sweat. I wash the bedsheets and yesterday's outfit, to see if the smell clears.

The flavour of things has also changed. Canada Dry ginger ale is revolting and tastes nothing like ginger ale. Hopefully I'll get those taste buds back in a few days.

The nausea is controlled but unpleasant. Yesterday, I crashed and had flu-like symptoms after the steroids wore off. When I feel that way, I should just nap for a couple of hours assuming my temperature is OK. It often coincides with more nausea which is also helped by napping. It may just be the new way my body has of telling me it's tired.

A memorial celebration

July 12, 2014

I've always liked wearing pink, but not breast cancer pink (or as my reiki healer today called it Pepto-Bismol pink). Since my diagnosis, I find it interesting the complete aversion many people have to the colour. I feel the need to announce, I'm not against pink, just please not Pepto-Bismol pink. I really like dark deep pinks as well as greens and blues.

On our yearlong bike-trip we had a bag stolen. Of all the things in the bag, the one loss that I felt the most was that of our mascot Puffie – a stuffed Labrador puffin that we bought at the L'Anse Amour lighthouse in Labrador. It got me thinking of memorials, and how they help deal with loss.

I crave a memorial for my breasts and wonder what others have done or if my ideas are totally crazy. On a couple of breast cancer social media groups, I receive a variety of suggestions for parties with catchy names (e.g., boob voyage) that all seem to involve booby cakes and lots of alcohol, which made me miss my girlfriends back in Ottawa. Those celebrations are more in line with *they've had a good life* celebration before they are cut off.

A fellow blogger who is probably about my age created an art piece the night before her mastectomy that touches my heart. I really feel for women who have children, whose emotional ties to their breasts relate directly to feeding their children as infants. I do not have that same bond but need to do something before my breasts are gone. Maybe it is just something trivial like swimming topless in Hawaii. (not sure its legal, but I'm sure an exception could be made). I now have photo shoot visions of Scott with the new Go Pro camera, taking pictures of me swimming topless with the sea turtles and snorkelling around the amazing coral reefs in Maui. Maybe we will even charter a sailboat to take us to a nice spot, not full of tourists. A place to say a last goodbye sounds like heaven.

Not without incident

———

July 13, 2014

My hands began to blister. Not just one or two blisters, but 9 on the left hand and least 4 on the right hand. They wake me up because I cannot spread my fingers nor clench my hands without pain.

The weakest time, known as nadir, should happen around days 8-10. In many people it aligns with the days where they are more fatigued. I will be extra happy to have my mother here to help ensure that I'm eating enough and getting out for at least a little exercise (although swimming, which sounds perfect, isn't advised when you have a higher risk of infection).

I call the on-call oncologist who doesn't think the blisters are chemo related. The location of the sores and my comments about allergic reaction send her on the wrong track. I take a couple Benadryl; however, the blisters continue.

It makes more sense to stop in at the emergency room at Stanford than drive home and call the oncologist again, who mentioned that I would need to be seen if the problem persisted. We want to check out the emergency procedures while I am happily ambulatory and not 'really sick' just in case I need the services later.

After five hours and consultations with the internal medicine resident, oncology resident, on-call oncology fellow, dermatology resident, and on-call dermatology attending (who happens to the be the director of oncology dermatology), I am diagnosed with a reaction to the chemotherapy called toxic erythema of chemotherapy. What put people off the diagnosis earlier is the atypical location of the blisters and the fact that I was doing so well otherwise. They were worried about Steven-Johnson syndrome (SJS), which would have been more severe and would have required IV corticosteroids.

We need to pick up some creams to help with these painful blisters. Unfortunately, the emergency staff sent us to a closed pharmacy. Back at home, I use ice and port numbing cream, which keeps me sane. Tomorrow morning, we can find the prescribed creams at a pharmacy. The medical team didn't change the chemo because the blisters are not considered a severe enough reaction to warrant a change.

Guilt

―――――

July 14, 2014

One of the ladies I talk to at a cancer group mentions that she is feeling a little like a 'chemo dropout'. She had a life-threatening reaction to chemo, and chemo was determined to be of marginal benefit. It was decided that she would not be continuing with chemo. There were several of us in the room just going through the first cycle of chemo, so she expressed feelings of 'survivor guilt'.

Another friend also went through the traumatic experience of having a tumour removed surgically, followed by reconstruction. However, in his case, the tumour had no cancer – so although he went through a lot of the same experiences – he isn't considered 'a survivor', because he didn't have cancer and that label, somehow, seems to be required. He lacks support groups and other infrastructure for those with cancer. While he is lucky to not deal with the constant fear of recurrence, he has survivor-guilt because he survived but wasn't as sick as others.

That comparison, that need to be part of the group, and yet the recognition that each journey is individual can prove to be a conflict. There will always be someone who has it easier, but also someone who has a much more difficult time. When we are together, there is a bond in that sharing experience, but also that twinge of guilt when you are doing better than someone else – also a lot of feelings of empathy – tearing at my heart strings – when I see others that are doing much worse – but also personal joy that I am doing well. Such a mix of emotions.

I'm feeling the pull of emotions right now as I enter my low blood count days aka chemo nadir. I'm looking forward to the rebound.

This too shall pass

July 16, 2014

At about 5pm, I felt these pulsing pains up my spine. By 8pm, they were excruciating whenever I was seated. Fortunately, I had a ride home. I could not imagine having to drive with this happening. I needed to be in the passenger seat with the seat partially reclined.

During support group, one of the ladies warned what the Neulasta bone pain felt like. With my blood count low (nadir), I'm also tired. The bone pain is caused by the Neulasta, which is a white blood cell booster. What is happening is that as the chemo leaves my system, my bones start reproducing white blood cells. My counts should rebound to almost normal in the next day or two. But the white blood cell booster means that my body is also suddenly producing an excess of white blood cells all at once. The bones go from not producing new blood cells (or producing them slowly) to having a sudden growth spurt and with that comes pain.

Sitting pain seems ironic, as I usually cannot work while standing as my arthritis gets in the way. Yet now I can only work while standing. I may also try going out for a walk, although it is a rather warm out. I wish I could swim, but with my blood counts low, that is not recommended. I am also in pain if I lay down in the wrong position. I need to be in just the right position to sleep. I'm waiting to hear back if my oncologist approves good pain meds. Unfortunately, Wednesday is not the best day to contact them, as my oncologists' nurse doesn't work Wednesday (there is someone that covers for her) and my doctor is on vacation this week, so to get that prescription the Wednesday nurse needs to track down the backup oncologist who doesn't know me.

If this happens next cycle, I shall be prepared! They don't give you much other than anti-nausea meds for the first cycle, and they wait for you to call. The idea is that everyone experiences chemo differently, so they don't know what you will need. They wait until they find out what you need and then prescribe it. At this point, it is all about managing the symptoms. Unless the problem is more life threatening than the cancer, the goal is to keep with the chemo regime on schedule through to the end.

Although Neulasta is recommended for the AC regime I'm on, many women opt to not take it. The clinical evidence is that it reduces hospitalization by 20% – however, if you are someone whose white blood cell count doesn't dip too low, then it is an unnecessary precaution. This is a medication that manages a side-effect of the chemo, and the side effects of the Neulasta can be worse than the chemo itself. It all comes down to deciding which is worse. Neulasta allows me to be more socially active. If I didn't take it, then I'd need to be a lot more careful about interacting with people during my low days, as my white blood cells might be a fair bit lower, and therefore my risk of infection higher. Since I need interactions with people for my mental health, it makes more sense for me to deal with the Neulasta side effects than it does for me to not take it.

My motto for today is, 'this too shall pass' ... although I'm also hoping the nurse calls back soon to tell me they have sent a prescription into the drug store for me.

In for an emotional day

———

July 17, 2014

Today, I get my head shaved. If you haven't done a chemo that causes hair loss you may not understand this idea of proactively shaving your head. Hair falling out in clumps is a pain. The second, more important reason, is it's an exercise in control. If I'm going to lose my hair, then I am going to control when it happens. Control is a huge issue with cancer, as it is one of the things you lose. You lose a lot of control over how your body is growing, how it reacts, and the various schedules of appointments. When you have an opportunity to take control and do something on your own terms, it can be important for some people. I'm a control freak and like to plan things. I struggle with my inability to plan our Hawaii trip because I have no clue how I will be feeling.

And so, I am taking control of my hair, and having it shaved today. Scott will get his head shaved too. We'll take a fun selfie when it is done! I'm looking forward to seeing what it feels like to have my head rubbed, the same way I like to rub Scott's head right after a haircut!

Things I love about a shaved head

July 19, 2014

I wonder if I will enjoy this as much when I'm bald as I do now. I am thankful that I look good with a shaved head. I only cover it up when I'm out in the sun to avoid sunburn. With nothing on, it feels like I'm wearing a hat all the time – the thin layer of hair seems to have the same sensation as wearing a tight skull cap.

I enjoy the feeling of the wind in my hair when I am in the car with the windows rolled down and almost want to stick my head out the window like a puppy dog! Unfortunately, I cannot stand the sounds of other cars, so this pleasure is reserved for when I'm driving on the back roads or side streets.

Petting myself by rubbing my hand down the back of my head never gets old – I catch myself doing it when stopped at a red light waiting for the light to change. I love the feel of the cold water on my head when I first jump into the shower after swimming. It takes a good 5 minutes for our hot water to reach the master bathroom. I used to make Scott shower first, as the cold water didn't bother him – now I'm finding that I enjoy it so much that I jump in first.

And of course, it's a lot of fun when Scott pets me too.

It's not a lump

———

July 20, 2014

My breast cancer pet peeve of the day is the word 'lump', because for me, it did not feel like a lump. The word lump is misleading and causes too many women to not get something checked out. It is part of why I waited a week. Fortunately, I only waited a week.Many women have lumpy breasts. Some of the normal tissue in your breast feels lumpy. It isn't the normal lumpiness that is the problem. It is the change that is a problem. The first I heard of nipple retraction was after I was diagnosed. What I noticed was a hard spot – an area that felt firmer than normal – which I initially associated with a muscle strain, but when it didn't go away, I got it checked out.

Get to know your breasts. I suds up with soap and feel around and inspect every time I shower. I also look at myself in the mirror and look down when I dry myself off. As a result, when something changed, I noticed.

The MRI image of my breast shows two masses. The upper is a known malignancy. This is the one I felt, and it is my largest mass. Depending on which scan, it measures somewhere between 3 and 4.7 cm. The MRI measured it smaller than the ultrasound, but they won't really know until they take it out and do a full biopsy on it. It is not a regular shaped nice round 'lump', rather it is an irregularly shaped mass. It doesn't look 3 cm in this angle; they base the size value on the largest dimension.

The bottom mass shows up on MRI only. I'm getting it biopsied tomorrow. It is suspected to be cancer only because I already have a known malignancy. The point I wanted to make with this picture is the irregular shape of my breast. I can visually see when I look in the mirror and while looking down that my left breast isn't smoothly curved. This is a sign that something is wrong.

It is cool that I can just sign a form and they mail me CDs with all the images from scans that have been taken. I get a full radiologist's report, so I know which images are most interesting as there are over 15,000 images from a standard diagnostic MRI.

Mouth sores and first cycle symptoms

July 20, 2014

I usually get canker sores when my iron is low, which also happens with chemo, so I was supplementing iron which kept the cankers to a minimum. True chemo mouth sores are nothing like a canker sore. They form on the side of my tongue, which apparently is particularly sensitive. Ouch.

I used a mouthwash that Scott made last night and this morning (and after anytime I eat) and the sores are starting to get better. I now know why the doctors ask, "Can you eat?", as the concern isn't the sore itself (that is a chemo side effect, and it will eventually heal). Their concern is that you are eating enough so that you stay healthy overall. Fortunately, among the odd prescriptions I got from my emergency visit (even the dermatologist was confused by this one) was a bottle of oral viscus lidocaine (like the dentist uses before putting in a needle), which is used to help provide symptomatic relief of the mouth sores to allow you to eat.

I've created a little chart for my oncologist (and myself to allow for planning next cycle) of my various chemo symptoms in the first cycle. I will use it when I next see the oncologist to get him to write in the preventative section at the bottom, such as when I should not swim, and any other activities I should be limiting at various times, as well as when I can and cannot take NSAIDs. I need the visualization to better understand things – and want to make sure that I'm not being too cautious about swimming, as it is something that I need for my mental health – especially if biking may involve blistering on my hands.

Seriousness is sinking in

―――

July 25, 2014

I'm starting to shed my hair. I noticed after the shower. There are enough bits of hair in the towel that I threw it in the wash!

At Wednesday's oncologist appointment, when I asked about surgery timing, specifying my desire to spend a week in Hawaii before surgery, the point was made not to push it too late. There is enough time for that week, but I should not plan on pushing surgery out 2-3 months. The comment was in the lines of, "We've done all this chemo, don't waste it". This cancer won't be killed that easily – even if the masses shrink to smaller sizes, they need to be removed.

Yesterday, I got a short synopsis of the pathology of the third small mass in my left breast. It is DCIS PR/HR+, HER2- with a small Ki-67 (<5%). This is sometimes called pre-cancerous or cancer in the duct itself, as it has not yet spread to the surrounding breast tissue. DCIS has a high likelihood of turning into IDC (which my other two masses are). So, this is my magic number three cancer.

Magic number three seems to be my meditation number. When I took swimming lessons last fall, the instructor had me breathe after every three strokes. Ever since then, three seems to be a better number for me when meditating. When I do yoga, I hold poses for three breaths, and when I try to calm my nerves to sleep, I count my breaths 1-2-3 and then repeat. Three seems to be my number.

Now that I have three unique tumours, it can stop there! No need to go any further!

Doing a triathlon before surgery likely needs to be rescheduled until after surgery. The window won't be long enough for me to manage it and Hawaii at the same time. Maui remains a plan since it is easy to get to and an easy island to get around.

These hurdles like to doing a PhD. At each phase there are additional hurdles to overcome. One bit of advice we are given in the PhD process is to celebrate each hurdle as you complete it. My first hurdle is AC chemo. I've done two treatments, so one could say I'm halfway, but that would not be fair, as I still need to recover from this second treatment before I can truthfully call it done.

I am happy to get some productive days back. My life isn't all about cancer anymore. I am re-emerging into my academic life, trying to pull together as much as I can to make a dissertation out of my existing thesis project. By fall, I shall have enough data to turn it into something. I have learned a lot and do have a lot to share – I just need to close it off and put it all together.

With the seriousness of this disease sinking in, what is also sinking in is my need to focus on the future – and on what comes afterwards or at least what I'm going to do with the next year and a half that doesn't involve chemo and cancer surgery.

Day three is just plain hard

―――――

July 26, 2014

Today is day three and it is a hard day. It was a hard day last cycle too. I am thankful that there will only be two more cycles of AC and that means only two more day-threes.

Why is day three so hard? The Neulasta pains are crazy. It is a different kind of muscle pain – pain from the inside out. It hurts to swallow but it isn't a sore throat. It is the muscles around the throat and the neck that all just plain hurt. And this makes me feel sad.

I walked this morning, and I even biked a short bit this afternoon, but that didn't seem to prevent the pains – although it was nice to get out – it is also very hot outside today – so I am thankful that we have central air. But it is still hard. I sleep and watch TV a lot.

The biopsy last Monday means I couldn't swim today. I missed my magical afternoon swimming with my clothing on. I will not allow anything to disrupt that routine next cycle as it is one of the things that helps me get through it. I'd also like to do reiki on day three, but my reiki healer is away this week, so I don't see her until Tuesday. Hopefully, she will be in next cycle.

Now I know, day three is hard, but it is just one day...tomorrow will be better.

There was a mix up on the schedule for chemo, so they had the wrong type listed for the second round. Now I know my last infusion date is set for November 17th. Surgery will be either December 10 or December 17. I need to decide which date to have them hold. That makes Hawaii the week of December 1st ... good news and something to look forward to.

What does it mean to be a survivor?

———

July 27, 2014

I don't know what it means to be a cancer survivor. I am a cancer warrior – I'm in treatment, I am living each day – but what does it mean to survive?

Some definitions involve the time after treatment when you are told you are 'cancer free'. This doesn't happen until after surgery when the cancer has been removed from your body. But I do not know, with breast cancer, when I will be considered 'cancer free'. After chemo, there will be surgery, after surgery there will be up to 10 years of hormone therapy. Am I cancer free after the surgery if I'm given the 'all clear'? Then the fight isn't against cancer itself, it is against 'recurrence' – which is an invisible devil. Is that when I become a survivor? Or am I a survivor if I remain cancer free after the hormone therapy? When do I get to start celebrating my 'cancer free' life?

I follow the blogs of a few women with metastatic disease. These women are fighters –everyday warriors – and I see them as survivors – as they have learned to live with cancer. For them, survivorship becomes more about a mental process – about how they see themselves. Each day that they fight, and live, they are survivors.

One of my fears is that I become a metastatic survivor – because the strength required to live with cancer is a lot greater than the strength to fight cancer. Chemotherapy is hard, and the entire thought of chemotherapy to slow the disease rather than chemotherapy to kill it is impossible for me to contemplate right now. I can fight this, because today I am a warrior and one day, I want to be a survivor.

Bilateral mastectomies

―――

July 28, 2014

A friend emailed a recent New York Times article about the prevalence of bilateral mastectomies entitled *The Wrong Approach to Breast Cancer* (Orenstein, 2014).

I read it with much interest but also much distain. There are several issues that are not addressed in the article, but it also highlights some important breast cancer treatment trends and issues. To make this discussion easier – BMX stands for bilateral mastectomy, and PMX stands for prophylactic (i.e., preventative) mastectomy.

The discussion is not about women with BRCA1/BRCA2 breast cancer genes. Some useful statistics: 12% of women in the general population develop breast cancer, of these, up to 5-10% (yes hazy statistic there) MAY have an abnormal BRCA gene. For this small percentage of women, the likelihood of breast (80%+) and ovarian (25%+) cancers is huge. Prophylactic surgery for these women brings peace of mind.

The New York Times article (Orenstein, 2014) highlights that PMX is unnecessary as it does not improve survival rates. The article highlights the over-use of this choice. What the article doesn't say is that one of the reasons so many women choose PMX is that they are sold on the ease of reconstruction. In the US, if a woman has breast cancer, insurance is required to pay not only for treatments but also for reconstruction. I was told this at my first surgical visit the same day I was told I had cancer. A woman from the UK commented that she was required to see a psychiatrist because she did not want reconstruction. The pressure to reconstruct is huge, but also, the way in which it is sold is misleading. The potential complications are understated.

The New York Times article talks about statistics but does not consider mental health. Most breast cancers occur in only one breast (I'm an oddity). In many cases, women have the first breast removed, but then choose the PMX for the second breast. In some cases, this is because of fear of cancer returning, as stated in the article, but in other cases it is because the women have difficulty living lopsided. The lack of symmetry becomes a constant nagging reminder of the cancer. It can be too much for some women. There are many women who are very happy about their choice of PMX and reconstruction, and many women who are happy about their choice for PMX and no reconstruction. What concerns me about this article is that research stated like this gives insurance companies a reason not to pay for the surgery, when it may be in the best interest of the individual. Mental health and quality of life after breast cancer are two variables that are not considered.

I'm concerned for women who have PMX because they are sold on the ease of reconstruction, but I'm also concerned about potentially denying PMX for women whose quality of life will be significantly improved by it.

My personal case is different. I don't qualify as a statistic in most studies because the nature of bilateral disease is not understood, but also because it is not very common. I have multi-focal cancers in my left breast (two tumours in different parts of the breast – the first is the one I felt (invasive ductal carcinoma, IDC grade 3 about 4cm), the second is DCIS (stage 0 non-invasive). In my right breast, I have about a 2cm mass IDC grade 2. It could not be felt and was found by a very good radiologist. For some unknown reason my body suddenly started to grow breast cancer quickly in multiple places. For me, the right choice is a BMX. It is not prophylactic, as I am not doing it to prevent a cancer from occurring. The cancer is already there.

I could have lumpectomies to remove the three areas – but then I would need radiation treatments. I would need to have mammograms and maybe even breast MRIs every 6 months for the rest of my life. I would need to go through biopsies every time they found something suspicious, and any shadow would be considered suspicious because of my history. I would also be so oddly deformed, with both breasts being different sizes and shapes which would present a constant battle with body image. This would lead to a terrible quality of life. I don't want to constantly worry about how I look or what will be said at the next doctor's appointment. It is bad enough to go through that during active treatment, I don't want that to be my life after treatment.

I love the idea of being flat and having choices. What I hope for most is that my breast surgeon does a good job and I have nice clean scars. Then I can choose to wear prosthetic breasts if I want an outfit to look a certain way, but I can also choose to not wear anything on a hot sunny day. I love the idea of a bra free life! To be honest, I rarely wear one now – but I'm finding that with all the biopsies and chemo insults to my breasts, I need to start wearing one more often, as they need to be supported.

What I really want to say about the New York Times article is that breast cancer treatment is an individual choice. Statistics can be useful in helping us make a choice, but the right choice is an individual one. For some women, a PBX is the right choice, even if there is no statistical advantage to it, for others it is not. I am insulted when the article assumes that women are making choices that are "not truly necessary" and assume that the doctor knows best, when the doctor isn't the one having to live with the decision.

Every day a new side effect

────

July 29, 2014

Chemo has many side effects, so many, that they don't tell you about them. What happens is, when you have a symptom, you contact your oncologist (or the oncologist on call) to see whether it is something you should worry about. There are so many side effects, many of which are rare or not that common, that listing them all to every patient would be impossible. But, from the patient perspective, I find myself constantly running into these odd side effects. I'm happy to be part of several face-to-face and virtual support networks. The virtual networks are useful for finding out whether something is "call the doctor immediately" or "pretty common, mention next time you are talking to your oncologist". My oncologist has mostly not been concerned about my side effects. Yet every day, something new pops up.

Yesterday's new side effect was loss of voice. Not a total loss, but suddenly my voice is hoarse, and it is more difficult to speak. This of course poses an interesting challenge, as I also have blisters on my hands from toxic erythema of chemo, which I also experienced last cycle. When the blisters are at their worst, typing can be painful, so I use voice-to-text on my computer. The hoarse voice makes that challenging. I don't know for certain yet if this is a chemo side effect or if there is something else going on, but my social networks tell me it is not uncommon. I just haven't yet had that confirmation from my oncologist.

I'm also losing my hair. Now, this is something that was expected, and it was why I shaved my head in advance of cycle 2. However, when people say that hair loss usually occurs on days 3-4 of cycle 2, I expected it to be a single day event. That isn't what is happening. My hair is getting thinner on various parts of my body. From the front, you don't notice the hair loss on my head (which made me think it wasn't happening), but from the back it is clear. It is also interesting to compare mine to Scott's, since we had them shaved at the same time. His is growing, mine clearly is not.

It is the towels where I notice it most. I've taken to using two towels after a shower, one for my head and one for my body – otherwise, I end up with the little hairs from my head all over my body!

Once the hand sores finish up, I prepare myself for the mouth sores. I'm now at a stage where food is tasting funny and my mouth feels fuzzy, like a layer of skin is shedding. Last cycle I had an annoying and painful tongue sore. Food finally tasted good, but it hurt to eat (ugh). I'm hoping that by using the magic mouthwash in advance, I can avoid the worst mouth sores this cycle.

Today was also my last swim until after my chemo nadir (blood count low). I have three days (8-10) where I cannot swim as my risk of infection is too high. I'll miss swimming, especially if my hand sores aren't healed as biking isn't an option when I have blisters on my hands. This also coincides with fatigue, so last time on day 10 all I did was sleep.

So far cycle two has not been as bad as cycle one because I have a better idea of what to expect. I can be more proactive about managing what is happening and plan my weeks out better. I now know not to commit to things on specific days, but on other days I can be more flexible. That helps. The control freak in me feels more in control.

The transformative power of a bike ride

———

July 31, 2014

I was sad getting out of bed after my afternoon nap. I had the energy to get on my bike and am in a strong phase. This felt like the kind of sad that looks a lot like depression – and that scares me.

I dragged my ass out of bed and had a bowl of ice cream. Chemo means I'm allowed comfort foods whenever I want them. And when I am sad, comfort foods help a little ... plus I knew I would need the energy, because if I was going to get off my ass and go for a bike ride, I needed to ensure my body was fuelled before I left.

I did it. I changed and hopped on my road bike. For the first half hour, I cried. My nose ran – most annoying side effect of chemo hair loss is that you lose the hair in your nose, so your nose runs a lot sooner when you cry. I allowed myself to cry. I contemplated anti-depressant medication. At some point, I will probably need it, but want to avoid the side effects.

About a half hour into my ride something changed – the endorphins kicked in – I suddenly started to see the beauty around me.

The bike ride transformed me – from sad-Becky back into warrior-Becky. For the remainder of the ride, I worked out the important arguments in a letter to the Editor for the New York Times that I plan to write (hopefully later this evening) relating to bilateral mastectomies.

I am still sad –just not dysfunctional sad. I've moved past that part and can now start to pull my thoughts back together into actions. I hope to get out for another ride first thing tomorrow morning before it gets hot and sunny, since I cannot swim tomorrow due to low blood counts.

My improved body image

August 1, 2014

Ever since my diagnosis, I have an improved body image. Sure, I am carrying a few more pounds than I would like, but I am proud of the way my body looks. I rocked the buzz cut! Now with my hair patchy and falling out, I find myself dressing up a lot more to go out. When I visit friends, or go to doctor's appointments, I wear nicer clothes and dangly earrings. I'm getting a bit obsessed about buying different things to wear on my head that (get this) complement the clothes that I'm wearing. I've never been that fashion conscious before.

But each day, I also read Facebook posts in the amazing Flat and Fabulous group about women who are afraid to walk outside after surgery. They are constantly worried about how they look and fight every day with negative body image because they don't want 'yet one more surgery' to clean things up. Some live in physical pain, while for others the pain is mostly emotional.

This worries me. I have never been happier with my body. I'm worried about what it will look like after surgery, but also what the surgery will do to my sense of body image. I want to keep this feeling I have now, and to always be proud and happy with my body the way it is.

Since the beginning of this blog, I've used the expression "my breasts are now public domain". I talk freely about them and posted an MRI picture of the cancers in my left breast. If I were back in Ottawa, I would be asking all my girlfriends to feel my left breast, so that they too would know exactly what breast cancer 'felt' like. As an educator, I am now in a position to educate people about what it means to have breast cancer. But I have to highlight that I'm an exception to the rule. My self-confidence and my current body image are not the norm. For too many women, this is an everyday struggle, and I find that sad. And every day I hope that surgery doesn't change my current body image.

Reflections on body image

———

August 3, 2014

While out walking this morning, my husband mentioned my body image blog post. He asked if it was because my focus is now on strength rather than fat or weight. Turns out my physician's response to my body was the biggest factor in my changed body image.

My family medicine (primary care) doctor says that I need to start considering my body weight. That I was starting to tip the scale from carrying too much weight towards obese. Yet, there was no focus on how strong I was or any other aspect of my physical health. I eat relatively healthy, and exercise perhaps a little excessively compared to the average person. Yet I never saw myself as being in good health.

Then my oncologist listed my health overall as "excellent". I was rather proud of that fact. Going into treatment for cancer I felt stronger and healthier than ever, so did not see myself as 'sick'. Cancer causes cognitive dissonance for me.

Upon reflection, I realize just how large an impact the view of my physicians has on my overall self-perception of my personal body image. Before cancer, I felt that I was overweight. Even though I was in good cardio shape, and strong (regular 30km+ bike rides), I still felt 'fat' and 'overweight'. I was 20-30 pounds over my "ideal" weight. I've lost 10 pounds and now feel much happier with my body the way it is. I'm proud of the classification of "excellent health" in my oncologist's records.

I think it is just interesting how much weight I put on the opinions (or perhaps the presentations) from my doctors and wonder what family (primary care) physicians might learn from this reflection.

My bald head

———

August 4, 2014

There are times when I find myself wanting to cover my head in something stylish – and I like looking good. There are times when I run to take out the garbage and cover my head so as not to scare or make anyone uncomfortable.

I usually wear my Tilley hat sailing, so anyone who has seen me before would not notice any difference. There was a moment when I took my hat off for a picture – because I really wanted a picture with the waves and my bald head – mostly for posterity. But I also wanted to feel the wind on my bare head. It was not that easy to put my buff and hat back on, as I needed my hands to hold onto the boat!

Towards the end of the sail, when it was a little less windy and cold, I found myself craving the chance to take off my hat so I could feel the wind on my skull. I love that feeling. But I didn't take off my hat because I was afraid of making others feel uncomfortable.

In the car, I often strip off my head scarf. It is either too hot, and I want to cool down, or I'm on a slower road and want to drive with the windows down. Again, that feeling of breeze on my bare skull is delightful. When I'm in the car, I'm not worried about how my baldness might make others feel (even when stopped at intersections). I'm conscious about it, but not worried about it.

I didn't worry when I had a shaved head and went out without covering up. But now, my head is mostly bald, with some patchy bits of hair. Sometimes when I swim, I don't worry about it and just go bare. Last time I swam, I wore my swim cap. I was OK with changing from my buff to my swim cap at the pool, and I even used the pool shower and exposed my naked head (but found myself hoping that when someone walked by that they didn't look my way). I didn't walk to or from the pool with a bare head.

I'm of mixed feelings right now. There are times when I want to look fashionable by using a pretty scarf/buff/whatever. The accessory becomes part of the outfit and dresses up what I'm wearing. However, there are times when I would rather not bother covering up. My bare head cannot be in the sun for any length of time, but my head craves being exposed for short periods of time.

How much should I worry or care about what other people might think, or about the discussions parents might have with their children after seeing me?

I bit the head off of the repair guy

August 8, 2014

I managed to get some real work done this morning, so it hasn't been a total write off. But every little errand tires me out. My body aches and I'm nauseated. When the repair guy called saying that he was at the front gate and wouldn't come find my apartment, but rather required me to walk out to the front parking entrance to get him, I already was not impressed. Then mid-way through repairing the microwave he sniffles and coughs. OMG. I freaked out internally and texted Scott, who suggested that I just ask him to leave.

My immune system is compromised enough that I was clear when the repair guy came last week that no one was to come if they had a cold. When he started to ask about the co-pay, which my landlord needed to pay, my brain was not functioning. I snapped and said, if you are sick, I need to you to leave because I'm having chemo and cannot be exposed. He clearly felt bad and explained that it was just allergies because the people at the last call had a cat. Since I still could not mentally process the co-pay issue, I called Scott and handed my cell to the guy. The repair guy politely went outside to deal with the issue and gave me the receipt when he finished.

I feel bad for snapping – but just couldn't manage it. It is frustrating that I can handle some mental tasks well, but others are beyond my abilities. I had the number for the property management folks someplace but did not have the capacity to figure out where that might be. I spent all morning working on getting my ethics submission for my thesis project – so clearly, I had some form of mental capacity – but this was just too much. My capacity for multitasking is pretty much gone.

Ugh, chemo brain!

My Buddha belly

August 10, 2014

I'm more scared that I'll look funny having a Buddha belly than I am about the flat chest from reconstruction.

I 'want' a double-mastectomy. Want is such an odd word here – need might be more appropriate. I do not want to be hacked up and left oddly deformed, which is what a breast sparing lumpectomy would do. I do not want radiation. My skin is so very sensitive that the idea of radiation burns freaks me out. So, for me, the best option is the double-mastectomy.

I do not want to go through 2-3 years of additional surgeries. When you are first diagnosed with breast cancer, the surgeon presents you with one bit of "good news": that insurance is required to cover reconstruction. They don't tell you that reconstruction is not easy. Reconstruction happens after they remove parts (or all) of your breasts, and then use radiation treatments to make sure that the cancer is gone. They begin reconstruction with less-than-ideal material – you are not starting with healthy breasts; you are starting with damaged breasts. The reconstruction process can (and usually does) involve several additional surgeries, all done under general anesthetic, bringing new risks of infection and complications.

Maybe if I had a small mass in one breast, I might opt for a simple cosmetic surgery that evens out my breasts – maybe. But I don't have that option. I have two areas of cancer in my left breast, one rather large, which doesn't leave much to work with. Plus, I have cancer in the right breast. Radiation would mean radiation on both sides – a double whammy.

For me, the best possible outcome is a single surgery – double-mastectomy with nice clean matching / symmetric scars. No extra lumps and bumps, but nice and flat.

What scares me is the Buddha belly. I have a great body image right now. I'm happy with how I look. I'm pretty sure I'll still be happy without breasts (they are trying to kill me after all). But the belly ... now that might be the challenge. I will need a new identity – perhaps after BCBecky (Breast Cancer Becky) I will become BBBecky (Buddha Belly Becky). Maybe if I can find some pride in that identity, I can be happy with my new body image. [I'm laughing through my tears as I write this].

Metastasis also scares me. So far, all signs are that I do not have lymph node involvement, but we won't know until after surgery. The first line of treatment for node involvement is chemo – which I'm already doing. The second line is radiation. If surgery finds node involvement, I may need radiation (ugh) and we'd look beyond the breasts for spread.

Women can live for years with metastatic disease (like 10 years). Metastatic disease is often treated with chemo that is designed to slow the spread of the disease, but the quality of life with sustaining chemo scares me. Chemo is hard. I can do it now, because I have hope that it means that when I'm done with chemo and surgery that the disease will be gone. I watch other women live with metastatic disease and go through chemo so that they can live a little longer, mostly to watch their children grow up. For them, the pain, the ugliness of chemo is worth it. I don't think I could do that. For the first time in my life, I truly appreciate what quality of life means.

I cannot see feeling awful from chemo just to live longer. I do not have kids or a reason to want to hold on. I could not bear to have Scott see me suffer for years just to live an unhappy life. I don't need to worry about it now. My prognosis doesn't look like that. From all signs I do not have metastatic disease, but these are thoughts that I do have ... and I promised myself when I started this blog that I would write these thoughts and share them, regardless of how difficult they might be to read or write.

Here is to living a long healthy life as Buddha Belly Becky ... whoever that may be!

This is what depression looks like

———

August 14, 2014

With the recent passing of Robin Williams, my Facebook and Twitter feeds filled with tributes but also warnings about depression. A friend posted a challenge to share pictures of people who suffer from depression as it helps to show the faces of depression. So, I took this picture today while out on my bike ride. One of the reasons I ride is to fight depression, but it is becoming more difficult.

Yesterday represented a transition (last night really) – from control to loss of control. I took the above picture in the middle of my ride. I cried for most of the first 30km. It wasn't until that point that I finally found myself back in control.

Fortunately, when I felt the early signs, I began to reach out, and I have my first oncology-psychiatrist appointment tomorrow and will be one of the first patients at a new oncology-psychiatry clinic at Stanford.

This is not my first bout with depression. Last time things were looking pretty good in my life and yet it was difficult getting out of bed in the morning. I slept more than 10 hours a day and had no motivation. I wasn't sad or anemic. I just wasn't motivated to do anything. That previous depression appeared as a lack of motivation rather than sadness.

On my bike ride today, I reflected on what I had learned about my earlier depression. I know which drugs worked and which did not. Uncertainty in life threw me off balance. Not knowing what to do after losing my job was a challenge. Relaunching a career wasn't a bad thing, but there were just too many of life's big changes happening in too short a period of time. My brain couldn't keep up.

This time it is about uncertainty, although my mom also pointed out that 'chemo-pause' might be a contributing factor. One of the side effects of the chemo drugs is a temporary onset of menopause. Young warriors call it 'chemo-pause'. In addition to the whole uncertainty associated with having cancer, I'm also dealing with emotions that may be enhanced by 'chemo-pause'. I'm thankful that people at Stanford understand the factors involved.

There is no certainty with cancer. Treatment is physically tough and the long road after treatment is emotionally and mentally tough. Be assured that I am well enough to know to ask for help when I need it.

AC cycle 4

―――

August 19, 2014

We had a three-hour delay seeing the nurse practitioner to sign off on chemo. Then we had an additional hour delay on the saline drip for rehydration. We arrived at the university clinic at 11:20 am and did not finish the infusion until after 7pm. Add in the 30-45-minute drive each way and it made for a long day.

I'm bound for Stanford again tomorrow morning for a recommended transfusion. My red blood cell and other vitals have been getting progressively lower with each AC dose. Any medication for low red blood count takes 6-8 weeks to work, and a blood transfusion has fewer side effects. However, I have some anti-bodies in my blood which means that the donated blood needs to be more closely screened to match my blood. The blood might not be ready – so we are to call first before driving up.

The new blood is due to come at a time when I usually have a low – so it might turn into a real blessing – giving me more energy when I typically don't have much. Crossing my fingers that they find a match before tomorrow morning.

Persistence, tenacity, and new blood

August 20, 2014

This cancer journey reminds me of when persistence and tenacity were needed to make it over that one last hill on our Going East bike trip. As Scott pushes the loaded recumbent bike up the mountain, you can see the sweat on his back. The locals thought we were crazy trying to bike over this mountain pass – but we were both persistent and tenacious and made it.

I feel like the entire road is uphill.

At my first blood transfusion yesterday, we were serenaded by a harp, which was nice. Med student- musicians volunteer to play in the cancer centre.

Now I have some new blood. I am still fatigued, but hopefully in the next day or two I'll bounce back :-).

Rethinking reconstruction

August 22, 2014

Yesterday, my oncologist gave me some good news when he said that my left breast felt like 'a normal lumpy breast' rather than a breast with a large cancerous tumour. This is a sign that the chemo is working. He also shared that we are on 'auto-pilot', finishing off the chemo regime with switching to weekly Paclitaxel (T-chemo) starting Labour Day for 12 weeks. Which gives me 12 weeks to figure out surgery.

I was so confident in my decision for no reconstruction, but that confidence was built upon what turned out to be incorrect assumptions. The surgeon reinforced my concerns about lumps and bumps. Since the reality is that I'm not a skinny girl, there is only so much a breast surgeon can do. Their priority is to remove the cancer and, with a mastectomy, to remove all breast tissue. Even with no reconstruction, I'm looking at two surgeries – the first to remove the cancer, and the second to clean up lumps and bumps. They cannot predict how I will heal. The surgeon strongly recommended a consult with plastic surgery and radiation oncology before I decide. Now I'm reconsidering my options.

If radiation is not necessary, then I'll be a strong candidate for immediate reconstruction. This would mean that during the same surgery I would have my breasts removed and a procedure done to replace my breasts with either an implant or some fat from another part of my body (usually the stomach). Breastcancer.org provides a good high-level description of the different reconstruction options. I'd rather go flat then have implants – in part because my body tends to react negatively to foreign objects, but also because they need to be replaced every 10-20 years. There are a couple of options that use stomach fat (not muscle) that may work out for me (DIEP Flap and SIEA Flap). I despise that the comparison chart advertises it as getting a bonus "tummy tuck", but in essence that is what happens. They move excess fat from your tummy and replant it in your breast – replacing the breast tissue with the tummy fat. If it works well, it gives a more natural look and feel as compared to implants – but the surgery time and healing time take longer.

The surgeon did a good job of encouraging me to think one year, five years, and beyond. I'm not suddenly going to become a skinny girl and will inevitably have various rolls and folds. Previously, I wrote a bit about my concern for Buddha belly. I need to consider what option is going to leave me with the best self-image? Since being diagnosed, I've enjoyed a positive self-image (more so than before diagnosis), but I don't know if that would still be the case after surgery.

The other thing that is often pointed out is that you do not know how you will react post-surgery. You may not think of your breasts as an important part of who you are now, but that might very well change when you wake up and they are gone. It's frightening. You could be 'certain' and wake up to discover that you were wrong. It's common to leave as many doors open for surgery. Rather than doing double-mastectomy with no reconstruction, they do a double-mastectomy with skin sparing techniques. The surgery takes longer, but it leaves you with more of your skin, making reconstruction easier. You can then decide later if you want reconstruction. This approach keeps the door open for options but also draws out the number of surgeries and the length of time you are being treated. If you make the reconstruction decision before the mastectomy and you are a good candidate, they can do the first two surgeries at once. That reduces the number of surgeries and overall healing time but increases healing time as compared to mastectomy alone.

Now I shall wait again, for the next set of consults, to see what my options are. Maybe I'll make a decision, but maybe not …

The regret test

August 26, 2014

My husband and I can be rather frugal with our money. This approach allows us to save, but also allowed us to take 16-months off work and bike around the world. It means that we have learned to always question when we buy something or spend money. We sometimes catch ourselves spending too much time debating over the cost of something trivial (like spending 45 minutes on the phone with t-mobile to figure out why I was charged $1.33 and getting it credited).

One of the biggest things that has changed since my diagnosis is that I often make decisions that involve spending money based upon 'the regret test'. What do I mean by that? I mean that I ask myself, 'will I regret not doing it?' If the answer is yes, then I worry a lot less about the cost of the thing.

What triggers my 'regret test' today is the thought of not seeing my father before going into my major surgery. My father cannot travel to me, so I need to make plans to travel to him. I booked us a trip to visit my parents in Canada during American Thanksgiving.

Queen of wishful thinking

August 29, 2014

When it comes to the entire surgery process, I am the 'queen of wishful thinking'. I had convinced myself that 'flat' was the way to go. In the 'Flat & Fabulous' Facebook group, I found that I was creating a new vision of myself that involved a beautiful flat chest – but it also involved a beautiful flat abdomen with no extra body fat.

I shall always carry extra body fat – if spending 16-months riding my bike around the world didn't cause the desired perfect 'flat' body, then why do I think that cancer surgery would fix this? I'm in great physical shape now, yet still have 40% body fat. I already eat right and exercise. As I age, I'm destined to gain a few more pounds, not lose them, and when you add in the early onset drug induced menopause that is part of the long-term treatment for hormone positive breast cancer, my weight battle is all up hill.

When the surgeon burst my bubble, I've had to seriously reflect: What do I want to look like after surgery? Long-term, what do I need my body to have a positive body image?

This last question is probably the most important. If my body image is tied to a lifestyle, then I most definitely need to ensure that I'm not setting up unrealistic expectations of myself. I should not expect that magically, after double-mastectomy surgery, my body fat will just suddenly reduce itself. The notion that I'll magically be transformed into this skinny girl with no breasts and an awesomely toned body – that is just me being completely unrealistic.

Realistic expectations of mastectomy with my body type would mean having a concave space under my arms where currently I have fatty breast tissue. Not 'flat' space there, rather concave space. Reconstruction would be required to put some fat there, otherwise, I'll have a gap between my armpit and my stomach fat where the ribs can be felt. My thoughts and focus had been on the front view, but I had not considered the three-dimensional view of my body.

I'm strongly considering the procedures that involve reallocation of my own body tissues as well as immediate reconstruction. This is a real option because I've done neo-adjuvant chemo, so the surgery will not delay chemotherapy. The only unknown variable is radiation. The surgeries that involve using my own tissue mean longer surgery (8-12 hours), longer hospital stay (4-5 days), plus longer recovery time (6-8 weeks). But from the reading I've done so far, I'm an ideal candidate. I have enough extra body fat, but not too much to bring an increased risk of complications. It will be interesting to see what the plastic surgeon says.

I'm in wait mode for a few weeks while I recover from my last AC chemo and subject myself to the first couple of rounds of T-chemo. The first two or three rounds are supposed to be the hardest on this new chemo, as your body needs to adjust to it. One step at a time!

Not talking = not writing

_____

August 30, 2014

Over the last few days, it has been extremely difficult for me to talk. I haven't done much over the last few days but watch TV and sleep, so I don't really have much to write or talk about.

My mouth sores got bad enough for me to ask for stronger drugs. I have been taking liquid morphine for the last couple of days – originally every 2-3 hours – but now I've backed off a bit. I slept through most of last night, which has gone a long way to helping me heal. Prior to that I was waking up hourly (or after morphine every 3-hours) with sharp mouth pain. The sore on the back of my mouth where the bottom of my tongue attaches is the worst. Simple things like eating, talking, even licking my lips are not possible. And the difficulty in clearing food from my mouth and brushing my teeth—Yikes! So many everyday things we do with our mouths. Who knew?

There is some improvement: I no longer feel like my tongue is too big for my mouth – it fits again. The roof of my mouth no longer feels like super scratchy sandpaper. Now it's more like the fine-grained black sandpaper.

I have a whole new empathy for those with severe chemo side effects. I can appreciate so much more how people find exercise to be a challenge (having not done any since Tuesday).

My excuse for not exercising has been an inability to hydrate enough. On Tuesday I rode my bike out to my eye doctor appointment, and I struggled with the heat and inability to suck water from my water bottle. The food I had brought with me to help keep up my energy stung when I tried to eat it. In addition to pain from motion, I found that I could not eat anything that was the slightest bit acidic or salty. Fortunately, after the appointment Scott picked me up.

Today I'm going to support group, knowing that few people are apt to be there on the long weekend, and I cannot really talk. It will be nice to see familiar faces and just be in the space with people.

Our bike adventure to take a train to downtown San Francisco and ride home is on hold. We may try it in a couple of weeks if the new chemo regime doesn't take too much out of me. These first couple of weeks might be difficult. Instead, tomorrow we will venture out to the coast for a walk on the beach. It has been a while since I've been out to see the ocean. I look forward to the smells and the sound of the rolling and crashing waves.

Short lived energy

September 4, 2014

My new sense of energy was unfortunately short lived. I was able to get a lot of work done over the last couple of days. I'll need to try to focus on reading an academic journal in the days to come.

Tuesday, I worked on a research ethics proposal. I felt rather productive, so it was a challenge to take a break and get out for a swim – but I needed the exercise. During my swim I felt strong. After my swim, however, I notice that my eyes were sore, and my face and neck were red. I had originally attributed it to using an ointment on my eyes the night before, but with further reflection it was likely a sun or the chemo reaction. I took Benadryl and slept well.

Wednesday, I woke up feeling kind of yucky. My stomach was unsettled, but I wasn't as nauseated as with AC chemo. I was low on energy yet managed a couple of short walks to the grocery store.

This morning, I woke late (after almost 11 hours sleep). I'm feel fatigued, but it isn't like before: it isn't relieved by exercise. Nerve pains are quite annoying and prevent me from sleeping. Random pains flash over my body, coming on like a pulse and then fading away. They are energy sapping. Tylenol makes the pains stop. Yay!

I don't know quite what is going on with my body right now, but I am definitely looking forward to getting my strength back. I'm still recovering from a difficult last week of AC chemo. I'd like to get back in the pool but I'm afraid to swim when the sun is out. I don't want to have another reaction. I'm hibernating for now, waiting for the sun to go down, and then perhaps I'll get out for a bit of a walk. I'm also waiting for a call back from the nurse, who might explain what these pains are and what can be done about it. This too shall pass...

A bike adventure

———

September 9, 2014

I haven't really said much about the Paclitaxel (Taxol) and various pre-meds side effects I'm experiencing.

One of the pre-meds is a steroid, which certainly leaves me feeling bouncy for the first two days. I'm trying to harness that extra energy by getting lots of work done and exercising. Last week, I was still feeling the effects of the mouth sores from AC and low red blood counts. Yesterday, when they tested my blood, it was almost at its lowest – so not surprising that I was fatigued most of last week. Today, I'm feeling a lot more energetic, but I cannot say if that is from the steroid or if it is a sign of improvement in the red blood count.

In the last chemo round (I'm now on weekly Paclitaxel infusions), I started feeling nerve pains on Wednesday, which got bad Wednesday night, were eased a bit on Thursday with pain meds but worsened with horrible joint pains and fatigue. Things were still problematic on Friday with nerve pain, joint weakness, overall fatigue, and some neuropathy. Overall, it wasn't a great week.

I'm waiting to see how things go this week. My first side effect (redness in the eyes, face, and neck) has been much less this week that last – so hopefully that is a sign that the side effects will lessen.

I hoped to get a 20km ride in today on my fastest, lightest road bike. I was cautious when I first started riding, and felt the weakness associated with the low red blood counts but also with a two week break in significant exercise. Once I climbed the hill onto the path, I felt pretty good – taking it easy, but enjoying the ride. When I got to about 7km, I felt that I might make my 20km goal. Then at just after 8km, I felt a thumping and thought there might be something stuck to my tire. I examined the tire, didn't see anything, tried to ride again but it was worse. After another examination, I noticed a sign of imminent rim failure. So I turned around but soon discovered the back wheel would no longer take my weight – I was destined to walk the bike home. Fortunately, my ride passes my house multiple times. I ended up walking almost 3km.

As I walked home with my bike, along the path, during the height of peoples' daily commute, I was struck by the sheer number of people who slowed down to offer assistance – more than 20 people slowed down and asked if I was OK in the 30 minutes I was walking on the path. One person even asked if I needed a spare tube. It is comforting to know that if I did end up with a flat on the side of the path, I would have no shortage of people willing to help me change my tire.

Insomnia and disrupted sleep is a Taxol side effect. I'm finding that through the first half of the night I wake up. I feel that I've slept for a long time but wake up to see only an hour has passed, and I have difficulty getting back to sleep. This repeats itself until about 3 or 4 in the morning, and then I seem to sleep for 2-3 hours. I may end up in bed for 10 hours, but only get 7 hours sleep. Last night I tried something different. I was wired up from the steroids, so rather than trying to sleep, I just stayed up and worked. I wrote a lot of blog posts and answered emails. I didn't go to bed until 2am, but unfortunately, I still found that I was waking hourly for the first part of the night. Today, with some exercise, we'll see if that helps with the sleep.

Cognitive numbness

———

September 10, 2014

I woke up feeling pretty good but have since experienced a cognitive decline. I ran a few errands which involved driving. I was fine when I first set out, but not doing too well by the time I got home about 90-minutes later.

After my bike adventure yesterday, I brought my wheel in for repair. Walking into the bike shop I noticed some numbness in my step, which is associated with neuropathy. On the drive home, my multitasking abilities were going and there was some mental separation between me and the world, almost a drunkenness. At this point, I make my way home and decide that I shan't be driving until this cognitive numbness fades. Even as I type, I have numbness in my hands. I had originally thought of it as neuropathy, but now I'm seeing it more as an overall cognitive numbness, rather than a tactile numbness.

I tell myself that now would not be a good time for making any major life decisions – or even doing any serious academic work. My mind is just not as sharp as it should be.

I still plan to go out for a bike ride. Exercise will do me good, and hopefully will help clear the brain fog. With my road bike out of commission, I'm going to ride my 'bent' today. I had a hint of some nerve pains last night before bed, but they haven't returned yet today. I hope they stay away. I want to get the bike ride in just in case the nerve pain starts again. If it hits as bad as it did last cycle, I won't be physically able to ride, so I must get out while I can. On the fatigue front, I'm not feeling the overwhelming tiredness I had at this time last cycle. There is hope that I am rebuilding my strength.

Definitely experiencing 'chemo brain' today!

Reflection on chemo brain

September 15, 2014

A great blog post by Anne Boyer (2014) crossed my twitter stream today. She talks about her experience with chemo brain after her first cycle of AC chemo.

I was lucky. I didn't have clear indicators of chemo brain during AC chemo – at least not until the last dose, at which time the mouth sores made everything else irrelevant. What I did have was an inability to multi-task or concentrate. If Scott played any music, I became unable to type, write, or think. My inability to multi-task began before chemo – as I had a hard time concentrating immediately after diagnosis (for that I blame stress and anxiety). However, I noticed during AC chemo that driving took a lot more energy. I could still do it, but to pay attention to so many things at once was exhausting. As the chemo progressed, I found myself thankful for the disabled permit that allows me to use a close parking spot at the grocery store. The cognitive effort associated with finding a parking spot would make running errands impossible. I need the disabled permit from a cognitive perspective.

As I venture into the T-chemo regime, my cognitive abilities are sharper for the first two days, and they then decline rather rapidly. I tried to blog about it, which in hindsight is rather remarkable. When I think about the experience and read t what I wrote, and then read Anne's description of the effects of Doxorubicin on the brain, I find myself wondering what are the effects of Paclitaxel on the brain? And what long-term effects will I discover of Doxorubicin (or not discover as I will have forgotten what I used to be able to do – a blessing I suppose).

I didn't mention in the cognitive numbness post the difficulty in describing something and not being able to get the words out. I pause while I talk. The language flow has somehow been interrupted. I hope that blogging is helping me with this since it gives me practice using my words. With each blog post I am exercising the parts of my brain that analyze and describe problems. This mental exercise may be just as valuable to my recovery as physical exercise.

I cannot help but be offended that these side effects are not talked about in detail. There was a brief mention in our "Introduction to Chemotherapy" workshop that chemo brain was a potential side effect, and that it was a real thing, and that it was being studied – but that is it. I find it offensive that this side effect has been understudied because women's description of the symptoms is often dismissed. This side effect is especially scary for me as an academic. When treatment finishes, will I still be able to do my work? I have a new-found respect for my friend who negotiated PhD courses while under the fog of chemo brain and while negotiating life in a new city. All I can say is Wow.

I haven't been able to read academic articles. Maybe it's a mental block unrelated to chemo. It might just be that my body wants to take a break from academic work and is resisting reading academic articles. I want to be more knowledgeable yet don't seem capable of searching for the right articles. I fill my 'high functioning cognitive days' with busy work. I get some contract stuff done. I catch up on my emails. I write lots of blog posts – but I don't read academic articles. I keep hoping that will change soon. I have a few articles starting to pile up in my 'to read' list ... I just need the cognitive presence and the motivation to make that leap – but it just isn't there yet.

For now, I shall keep up my exercise and try to write regularly. I can only hope that my words continue to make sense and continue to demonstrate some level of cognitive competence.

I'm scared

September 17, 2014

I have given myself permission to go into surgery kicking and screaming. I'm OK with not being calm and collected when I get rolled into surgery. It is natural to not want to deal with it.

What has me scared today? I went for a bike ride and the exercise seemed to make the neuropathy worse! Unfortunately, my 18km ride today will likely be my last ride on my road bike until after T chemo – unless something changes. I'm further off the ground than on my recumbent and feel disoriented and like things move too fast. The bike is less stable – so more risk of falling. I shall miss it, but alas, it may be time to start looking into indoor exercise options.

On Monday, when my oncologist mentioned that if the neuropathy gets too bad, we stop the chemo and move up the surgery date – that scared me. I have things planned – I have plane tickets booked. I don't want to have to change my plans ... I want to continue to feel like I am in control of this process ... so today I'm scared. Scared that my well laid plans will all need to be tossed to the side as I deal with this disease ... ugh.

Thanks for the hugs

September 18, 2014

Thanks for the emails and virtual hugs after my post yesterday. I really appreciate the support. Often when I get into one of my down moods, I just need a little encouragement.

I tend to 'catastrophize' by imagining the worst possible scenario and am especially prone to this type of thinking when I'm not feeling physically well. The first step to stopping it is to recognize that it is happening. It wasn't long after I posted I'm scared that I realized that my brain was stuck in a worse-case loop and not moving beyond that. Once I realized it was happening, I changed my thinking.

Although I'm feeling neuropathy and pain, there are ways to manage it. The worst of it is limited to about 12-72 hours depending on the cycle, and for the most part, things clear up before the next cycle. Stopping Paclitaxel is not a consideration yet. We'll cross that bridge when we come to it.

I've now processed the things that I was worrying about. We can deal with the wrenches in the path when/if we need to.

It is important to write about my feelings when they are happening – even when they aren't happy comfortable feelings. If I don't write about my down days, I'm not being honest about the journey – but also, others who read my blog need to hear that down days are a normal part of this process too.

Today I'm doing better. Thanks for the hugs.

Grumpiness

September 22, 2014

I was grumpy by the time we made it into the infusion centre. I waited an hour after my appointment time before I got a chair – they were out of chairs and beds, so I had to wait until one cleared. Then, when I got one, it was in the corner – it feels like I'm tucked away. The person beside me had the curtain drawn so I felt like I was in a little cave. I was already grumpy, so waiting an extra hour and getting a yucky spot didn't make me happy.

Then the order in the system was wrong. It showed the amount of steroid I was on for cycles one and two (20mg) instead of the change we made last cycle (8mg). We managed to get the nurse to let me take 8mg while we wait for the callback from my oncologist (the nurse checked with my oncologist's nurse practitioner). Because I take the steroid by pill, I need to wait 30 minutes after taking the steroid before chemo – so waiting for the callback and then having to wait another 30 minutes was trying my patience.

Honestly, I'm just tired of the chemo routine. The last few weeks I've had more bad days than good days. I keep hoping for a rebound, but it isn't coming as quickly as I'd like. After today I will be one third of the way through Paclitaxel. I can't wait for this to be done!

Pathological complete response

———

September 23, 2014

I've been reading about the expected pathology reports for post-mastectomy after neo-adjuvant chemotherapy. That is, what should I be hoping for in the pathology after chemo – and what does that mean?

"Pathological complete response" or pCR –indicates the degree to which the chemotherapy treatment has killed the cancer. According to (Cortazar et al., 2014), you are considered to have a pathological complete response if:

- absence of invasive cancer or in-situ cancer in breast or the axillary nodes (ypT0 ypN0)
- absence of invasive cancer in breast or axillary notes but in-situ is present (ypT0/is ypN0)
- absence of invasive cancer in breast but in-situ and nodal involvement (ypT0/is)

The research says, that for the type of tumour I have, if I have a pathological complete response. then it is a good indicator of my overall survival. The studies don't say anything about survival if you don't achieve pathological complete response. The purpose of the two studies I looked at was to determine when/ if pathological complete response was a good indicator of disease-free survival. The answer for my type of cancer is yes – if the pathology comes back with pCR then that is a good indicator of disease-free survival.

I now know what I should hope for when the bilateral mastectomy surgery pathology comes back.

I now really want to know the pathology from my bilateral mastectomy before committing to the DIEP flap surgery. This has me leaning towards a skin sparing mastectomy with immediate reconstruction with tissue expanders, which means that if I want the DIEP surgery later, I can have it. Or I can have the expanders removed and skin cleaned up if I don't want it. It leaves the door open for reconstruction or not – and the decision will likely depend on prognosis. If I'm going to live a long healthy life post breast cancer, then the DIEP surgery is a worth-while investment in my time and physical energy. If the prognosis is not so great, then I'd rather be done with the surgeries and get on with living.

Reconstruction update

—————

September 26, 2014

I really liked the plastic surgeon. This is good.

We walked through the different surgeries and options. She validated that I'm a good candidate for DIEP/SIEP reconstruction based on physical exam. There is another test that she will order – a CT of the belly – to see whether my blood vessels are big enough to allow for the surgery. I hope that December 17th still works with the schedulers. It is a challenge to schedule this surgery as it is an all-day event for the plastic surgeon (8–10-hour surgery) in addition to requiring the breast surgeon.

The go/no-go on this surgery will be determined by scans done at the end of November, before the next surgery consult. At that point, scans are done to see just how well the chemo has worked. This will be the best information we have prior to surgery.

The plastic surgeon helped me better understand and feel more comfortable with both the surgery itself and the recovery. Regardless of whether radiation is required, the option that is likely to have the best outcome both aesthetically and recovery wise is to do the reconstruction immediately (so with the BMX). From her perspective, I am healthy. I don't have other illnesses that would increase my risk of complications.

I'm amused at how she looks at my body and wants to sculpt it – to reshape it – and how she casually mentions a revision surgery that involves liposuction to remove various extra fat bits allowing for a better cosmetic outcome. She comments that you don't realize the fat is there until after the first surgery – you become more aware of different fat pouches after they remove the belly fold. I cannot help but feel pleased about this potential sculpting, but I'm also cautious. It is not a surgery that I would choose if it wasn't for cancer.

Somehow, I feel a lot calmer and less anxious. Surgery seems more like something that I can handle and recover from.

I feel a little calmer at the idea of looking down after the surgery and seeing myself – if they are able to spare the skin and nipples (they only do this if the various in-surgery biopsies are clear) – then when I look down it will look like me. My outside will be the same, the inside will be different – but it will still all be me. With less belly, my hips will look huge. Instead of difficulty fitting shirts, I'll have difficulty fitting pants. This doesn't bother me. I can imagine myself looking sleeker – feeling good about my body.

I've been replaying the diagnosis in my mind. I don't know why. I keep going through that day in my head – the day everything changed. Today I'm able to see beyond chemo and even beyond surgery – and that is good.

This decision feels right.

Engaged patient in a hospital gown?

September 27, 2014

Since my diagnosis, I've seen many different specialists: breast surgeon, medical oncologist, chemo dermatologist, and plastic surgeon. My doctor's appointments have gone something like this.

Medical assistant takes my vitals.

Medical assistant directs me to remove clothing usually waist up and put on a gown opening in front.

I wait 10 minutes or up to 2 hours for the doctor.

Doctor comes in and talks to me for 10 minutes to over an hour depending on the type of appointment.

Doctor examines me for 1-5 minutes.

Appointment ends and then I get dressed.

I remember how at the first appointments, I felt awkward talking to the doctor while I was undressed. It was odd that the doctor would do the entire consult/ discussion (with appointments that were 30+ minutes involving a fair bit of question and answer) while I was undressed. I wonder if this is an oncology thing or an American thing? It wasn't until a friend mentioned it, that I realized the power dynamic at play here. By being the patient, I'm already in a lower 'power' position in the healthcare system. By having me remove my clothes, that just increases the imbalance (or ensures the imbalance is maintained). It isn't conducive to a collaborative dialogue, nor does it encourage me to be engaged.

In the Canadian primary care setting, the doctor first comes in and talks to me, then steps out so I can undress and put on a gown. During the examination we talk a little bit before the doctor leaves again to let me change. Any needed further discussion happens after I'm dressed. There are never those awkward moments where I'm sitting in a hospital gown, trying to ask questions and absorb all the new information.

At Stanford, I now bring a hoodie that zips up the front. After changing, I put my hoodie over my gown. I can comfortably ask questions while sitting in the chair (not on the exam table). The hoodie helps me avoid feeling exposed and cold and is easy to unzip for the exam. Doing this helps me feel a lot more empowered and comfortable.

I cannot help wondering why the system is this way. It may save time, but really, given the back-and-forth, especially in a teaching setting, it doesn't make a difference. Perhaps this is just a legacy practice from when the patient's feelings were not considered. With the push to have engaged patients, perhaps we need to start rethinking these processes with the patient in mind?

Not your stereotypical surgeons

September 30, 2014

Surgeons get a bad rap for being insensitive and un-empathetic. From the outside, they are seen as the engineers of medicine – socially awkward, mechanical in their interactions, and having no time for patient engagement.

This has totally **not** been my experience. I have seen a couple of breast surgeons, a couple breast surgery fellows, a plastics resident, and a plastic surgeon. The surgeons have been highly empathetic and spent a large amount of time educating me on my surgical options, which seems to be part of the learning process.

In my experience, attending surgeons are most empathetic. The residents are still learning, so their interactions can feel a little mechanical – they are still trying to figure out the best ways to make connections with patients, but also the best ways to describe things. By the time they are fellows, there's a higher level of confidence in their ability to provide patient education. You start to see customized information for each specific case.

The best early advice I received was to 'decide who you wish to trust' in treatment. In the first couple weeks after diagnosis, I decided where to get treatment based on where I felt comfortable – but also had the most options. I really liked being in a teaching setting and having access to more specialists – but that was balanced with knowing that I would spend more time in waiting rooms and receive less fancy care (e.g., the infusion treatment centre doesn't provide lunch).

After a couple of appointments with my breast surgeon, I decide she is someone I wish to trust. After my first visit with my plastic surgeon, where she spent over an hour talking to us, she too becomes someone that I trust. Deciding to trust allows me to filter through a lot of additional information and advice. It allows me to be OK with the decisions I'm making and be a lot more comfortable with my upcoming surgery.

Society gives surgeons a bad rap but at least from my experience – the breast oncology and breast plastic surgeons have been awesome so far.

The generosity of strangers

October 5, 2014

If you have read this far you are now aware that I'm an avid cyclist. Cycling has been one of the things that kept me sane though AC chemo and one of the things I've struggled with on Taxol. One of the unfortunate side effects of Taxol is cognitive disassociation – where my brain cannot process visual cues as fast as it normally does. I've had to stop driving. Until my last chemo cycle, I was able to drive a couple of days a week. Now I'm not comfortable driving at all. In addition to not driving, I've also been challenged with biking. The biggest concern is that my balance isn't what it used to be. In addition to not processing the visual cues, I'm also not as solidly balanced on my bike. Unfortunately, I've come to a point where I can no longer ride any of my bikes.

Fortunately, there is the internet and I'm connected to various communities. I posted a plea to a recumbent riders' community. One of the folks came to my rescue. This afternoon, he dropped off his Trident Tadpole Trike for me to borrow while I'm on chemo and recovering from surgery, as I will not be able to put any weight on my arms. Tonight, I got a chance to take it out for spin. It was a hoot to ride. I'm so happy to be back on a bike again. Unfortunately, the front wheels are slightly too far apart, such that it doesn't easily fit through the front door. I can only ride when Scott is home to bring the bike in and out for me. I'm not currently strong enough to lift it, although that will change when I stop chemo and regain some of my strength. For now, I'm just happy to be able to get out and ride a few days a week.

One more chemo day

October 6, 2014

I've survived one more chemo day. I type this as the monitor beeps saying I'm done. With any luck this will be my last infusion.

I won't know until next Monday, which also happens to be Canadian Thanksgiving, what is happening with my chemo. I have an MRI on Thursday night and various doctors' appointments on Monday. If the tumours are gone or small enough, then we will stop chemo and get ready for surgery. If the tumours are still present on the MRI, or haven't shrunk as much as we had hoped, then I'll continue with chemo for another six weeks.

This means another week of appointments. I'm going to try to take it easy this week – listening to my body – and doing whatever I feel like doing. Pretty much like I have been doing since starting chemo with a little more emphasis on resting.

I'm now having pain under my nails on my thumbs and first two fingers. Even when typing, I'm aware of the pain. The fingertips are sensitive to heat – in particular the heat of the gas burners on the stove. I'm going to try to shift to meals made in the oven.

Oh, where has my mind gone?

October 8, 2014

In one moment, I feel like I'm thinking clearly. I'm reading and reflecting. I feel connected.

The next moment, I realize just how unconnected my mind is. This chemo brain is infuriating! I ventured out today – unable to drive because of the cognitive dissonance that is getting worse with each cycle. I took the local train to the mall to buy a ridiculous amount of chocolate. I treated myself to a 30-minute reflexology foot massage (hoping that it might help with the neuropathy). I failed to turn off the stove when I made breakfast this morning. I'm perfecting the poach egg – just need to learn to turn the stove off after taking the egg out of the pot! Fortunately, I didn't do much more than burn the bottom of a pot.

I have several blog posts in the works. In the times when I'm thinking clearly, I reflect, and write. I seem to be OK when I'm sitting in front of my computer – with that limited field of vision. But when I step outside to walk, visual processing is a challenge. I find myself looking down at the ground as I walk, mostly because I cannot process what I'm seeing when I look up. It is confusing. My vision is also getting worse. It doesn't help that my vision was all screwed up from cataract surgeries even before the cancer. But the chemo is changing my vision, so my glasses aren't as clear and my eyes without glasses aren't working well.

I'm so looking forward to being done with chemo!

My first Pink'tober

October 10, 2014

October is a month full of tacky fundraisers in the name of breast cancer awareness. I didn't really notice Pinktober before. It had no meaning in my life.

Now, I cannot help but be aware of Pinktober. This is cause-marketing, where companies partner with breast cancer charities to raise money for mutual benefit. Some are good; however, some are downright tacky. Diane Mapes over at Double Whammied wrote a great satire piece on what other cancers might look like if they were advertised the same way as breast cancer *What if people treated other cancers like they do breast cancer?* (Mapes, 2014). She helps to elucidate the over-sexualizing found in many breast cancer awareness campaigns.

A lot of money is raised for good charities during the month of October, but I am still bothered by the advertising. The one I keep seeing on TV is the 5-hour energy fundraiser for Living Beyond Breast Cancer (http://www.lbbc.org). I've attended an online webinar by LBBC on chemo brain that was very useful. They do some good work. However, I was bothered by the video clip because they didn't show anyone young, which didn't speak to me in any way. I would support Living Beyond Breast Cancer, but not by buying a 5-hour energy drink.

I was particularly incensed by the fracking company painting its 'bits' pink (Abrams, 2014) in a publicity stunt. Who thought that was a good idea? Many in the blogosphere (Lurie, 2014) thought it was a spoof. It is one of the more blatant pink washing examples.

Many awareness campaigns are mostly sexualizing breast cancer, and that sucks. Frankly, breast cancer sucks. Over the years I have had friends diagnosed with other types of cancer. They were told "if you are going to have cancer, this is a good one to have". No one ever told me that, and rightly so. If you are going to have cancer, breast cancer wouldn't be my first choice.

Now I get the pleasure of living through October, having to be constantly reminded of the ugliness of breast cancer, and watching misguided *awareness* campaigns that make it even harder for young women with breast cancer to have a positive body-image. Here is another misguided campaign – I love boobies (Foundation., n.d.). It pretty much sends the message that those of us with breast cancer didn't take care of ourselves, that we are now freaks because we no longer have boobies.

As someone living with breast cancer, one of my biggest fears is how this is going effect my body-image – what I feel about my body. I haven't had surgery yet. One of the scariest parts of surgery is worrying about how I'm going to feel afterwards. Not the physical part, but the emotional and mental part. I think this is because I haven't yet internalized the "my breasts are killing me" message. I'm still dealing with "chemo made me sick", rather than "cancer made me sick".

Although I'm in favour of breast cancer fundraising to support women living with and beyond breast cancer and those who are funding research, there is such a thing as positive (win-win) cause-marketing. Partial messages and ad campaigns make those of us living with breast cancer feel worse. There should be some kind of cause-marketing rule: they should be talking to people living with the disease and be more sensitive to the real struggles of the disease.

Please stop telling me how much you love your boobies, because I'm not going to have mine for much longer!

Mentally preparing

―――――

October 12, 2014

I am preparing for disappointment. I can endure six more rounds of chemo, but only if I can have a week off to gain some strength. Love how I'm bargaining with this cancer? Tomorrow I'll be bargaining with my oncologist. I only hope that taking a week off is possible and makes sense. If I have a week to regain some strength, grow a few more red and white blood cells, and allow my mouth sores to recover, then maybe I can endure six more weeks of this chemo.

I will be pleasantly surprised if the MRI comes back saying that the tumours are gone or even mostly gone. This would mean that I stop chemo and start regaining my strength in preparation for surgery. As much as I'd like this option, it isn't what my gut is currently telling me. When I bend over, I can still see some skin retraction – so I can still tell where the larger tumour was. It no longer feels like a hard spot – and the doctors say that my breasts feel normal – but I can still see signs of it. This could just be scar tissue or dead tumour remnants.

I'm mentally preparing myself ...

Groundhog Day

October 13, 2014

Thinking of Groundhog Day: if the groundhog sees his shadow, then 6-more weeks of chemo. If he doesn't see his shadow, then we are done with chemo. Today is mostly cloudy (figuratively, not literally, it is almost always sunny here).

MRI results are rather encouraging, although I don't completely understand them. There is no sign of nodal involvement. The more encouraging line relates to the large tumour on the left breast (L1): "there is near complete resolution of abnormal enhancement". The other two tumours, L2 and R1, have shrunk but are still there. These were slower growing. It isn't surprising that they are less responsive to the chemo. The consensus is that I've had an excellent response to chemotherapy and that I can proceed to surgery at any time. Chemo is only needed until surgery. If they cannot get the surgery scheduled soon enough, then additional chemo is needed.

The breast surgeon recommends a two-stage approach – the first being a lumpectomy, sentinel node biopsy (axillary lymph node dissection only if positive biopsy), and de-vascularization of the nipple and areola complex. All the removed parts are then sent to pathology for full analysis. In essence, this is the cancer surgery plus de-vascularization of the nipple area. The de-vascularization increases the blood flow to the skin around the nipples, reducing the risk with the reconstruction. It also includes a biopsy of the area under the nipple, which determines whether the nipple can be kept. This is done approximately three weeks after the stop of chemo. I'm waiting to hear on dates for this.

The second surgery is bilateral mastectomy sparing the skin and nipples (only if they are cancer free) with immediate flap reconstruction. This happens about three weeks after the first surgery. This is tentatively set for December 17 but will likely be earlier.

What I like about this approach is that we get the cancer out quickly – so it is gone before it gets a chance to grow again. We will also have the pathology report before reconstruction. It doesn't necessarily change the surgeries, but it is a consideration. Having confirmation that radiation isn't required makes the breast surgeon's part of the second surgery a little easier, but that isn't the big part of the second surgery. The bigger part is the reconstruction – so the second surgery is still a long surgery (8-10 hours).

After the second surgery I start hormone therapy (tamoxifen) for 10-years. They call it hormone therapy, but what it really does is remove the hormones, so it is more like anti-hormone therapy.

There is also a third surgery that takes place no sooner than 3-months after the reconstruction. This is the "revision" surgery. Once everything has healed from the cancer surgery and primary reconstruction, the plastic surgeon goes back in and cleans up any scar tissue and liposuctions any extraneous fat pockets.

Where does this leave me? After all the surgery discussions today, my oncologist still wants me to do one more chemo treatment. I wasn't willing to do it today due to mouth sores that need a little more time to heal. I have chemo on Thursday. Depending on when the first surgery date is, this will likely be my last chemo.

Temper tantrums

———

October 15, 2014

Yesterday, I felt like a two-year-old having a temper tantrum. **I don't wanna!** I screamed to myself as tears dripped down my eyes.

I got a call from the surgery scheduler. They were awaiting word from my oncologist about chemo scheduling. After conferring with my oncologist, I got word that the plan is to do chemo on Thursdays until the end of the month, do the first surgery on November 19, and the second surgery on December 17. This, in theory, is the plan – however, I have not yet received confirmation on anything other than chemo this Thursday – which was the "one more" my oncologist and I agreed to on Monday. I knew there might be more than one more, but I don't have to like it. My one goal on Monday was to not have chemo on Monday – I just need a couple more days to feel better before facing any more. I've been glad for these last couple of days.

I'm of quite mixed emotions. This plan works for me – it lets me still get in a trip to Hawaii before the first surgery, and a trip to visit my parents before the second surgery. We ran through the schedules last night, and it even looks like my friends from Nova Scotia can still join us in Hawaii (yay). The extra chemo gets me that much closer to finishing the protocol (which calls for 12 sessions of Taxol – in the end I'll have 9 sessions).

Part of me doesn't want the extra two chemo sessions – I'd just like to stop chemo and go on with the surgery, but what if those extra two are the difference between beating this thing and not? Will those two extra sessions be extra insurance against recurrence? Metastasis? Of course, we have no way of knowing whether or not a couple more sessions of chemo will make any difference whatsoever. But to align with the surgery schedules, it is best that I am in chemo right up until three weeks before surgery. And then I get four weeks between the first surgery and the second surgery. I'm happy for a little extra time to ensure that I've healed.

The two-year-old in me is jumping up and down screaming about the need for more chemo, but the logical side of me is OK with the new plan but would like to see some form of confirmation on the new dates, so that the planner in me can make travel arrangements!

Chemo and an update

October 17, 2014

Yesterday (Thursday), I had my 7th infusion of Paclitaxel (Taxol). Thursday was my Star Trek Voyager treatment (7 of 9).

I now have my last two Taxol treatments scheduled for Thursdays. Next week it'll be neat to go to a different, newer infusion centre because they couldn't get me in at the regular place. My last session (Oct 30) is at the normal infusion centre because I need to hear the chemo song and say farewell to all the wonder chemo nurses there after 13 treatments (4 AC, 9 Taxol).

My two surgery dates are confirmed. The first surgery will be on November 19. One nice thing about this schedule is that we were able to rebook our Hawaii trip from December 3-11 to November 10-17. I'm so looking forward to that trip.

I have clearance for traveling the week after surgery. I scheduled a trip a while ago to visit my parents and it is back on for American Thanksgiving. I'll have a checkup with the surgeon on Monday November 24 to ensure that I'm OK to fly. The expectation from the surgeon's office is that it won't be a problem.

The second surgery (the long 8-10-hour surgery) will take place on December 17.

I have a lot of appointments scheduled – to talk about the details of the surgeries and the details of the pathologies. I'll end the year, December 29th with an appointment with my surgeon to hopefully remove drains, and oncology to go over the full pathology reports. It is at this point where I hope to get the message that I'm free of breast cancer (NED – no evidence of disease). That would be a very nice way to enter the new year.

Reclaiming pink

———

October 18, 2014

An acquaintance with metastatic disease is having a personal fundraiser and, in her invitation, she talked about 'reclaiming pink'. This reminded me very much about the work we do as Unitarian Universalists of reclaiming religious language, a message that resonated very strongly with me and allows me to call my local congregation a "church" even when I don't identify as a Christian. There is power in taking back language and symbols that have been co-opted by others for not so altruistic purposes. I like pink. I often wear pink. I don't feel a visceral need to avoid pink. But now that I have breast cancer, pink is a loaded colour. It has a message in it, and in that message is power.

I've blogged recently about *My first Pinktober*. What do I want to do for breast cancer awareness? Blogging about my experience with breast cancer is what I can do for awareness. I want to also re-claim pink by getting a pink t-shirt that says something like: *Ask me about breast cancer* - maybe with a pink ribbon and my blog address.

Ask me about breast cancer is an invitation to talk about it, which is a key for part of awareness. Of course, I'd only wear it when I was willing to have conversations with strangers about it, which is pretty much most of the time. It would allow me to reclaim pink to support the message I want to support.

Now I just need to figure out how one gets the custom shirts I want made.

Learned helplessness and patient engagement

October 20, 2014

My oncologist has a new nurse, and I sure do miss the previous nurse. The new nurse doesn't answer my electronic messages through the secure *My Health* system in a timely fashion. The original nurse checked at least twice a day. I often had a reply within hours of messaging. We had an understanding. I emailed my concerns and she replied the same day. There was no need to call. I only called if the issue was urgent (e.g. I needed pain meds the same day). Now I feel like my messages are going to a void. I report a new side effect or problem, and I wait. After at least 24-hours I get a response. I can no longer expect a same day reply. Sometimes it takes 2 days – which is an eternity when you are waiting on pain meds or trying to proactively treat a side effect.

I have developed a mild form of learned helplessness. Since reporting was not making a difference, I stopped reporting. My behaviour as an engaged patient changed because of a healthcare team behaviour change.

What is important in this observation, is that when healthcare providers want patients to 'comply', the providers need to do their part in acknowledging that compliance. If you want me to report my side effects, you need to acknowledge them when I do report. Otherwise, I feel like I'm wasting my time and energy.

Another important note here is that you don't necessarily need to solve the problem. As a patient, when I'm having a chemo side effect, I sometimes just need a little re-assurance and that what I'm feeling is OK. It happens. It isn't a serious complication. I just need an acknowledgement. I want you to note the side effect in my file, so that when we discuss my care at the next appointment, you have a better picture of my experience. I believe I am doing my part to help ensure that you have information about my experience, to help you recommend care that aligns better with my needs. It is a partnership – but that partnership only works if you acknowledge my attempts to communicate with you.

Learning to assert myself

_____

October 29, 2014

Today, I asked for a supervisor.

The online system showed my appointment as 9:15. I was told to arrive 30-minutes prior to my appointment (which is a bit excessive). I arrived 25-minutes prior to my appointment (8:50). When I was still waiting at 9:30, I talked to the receptionist. Anytime I'm asked to wait more than 15-minutes, I want to know why I'm waiting. That is a lesson I have learned here in the US. In Canada I would just wait in silence. It is interesting how asking goes against my ingrained behaviour. I found out that my actual appointment was at 9:45. The online system had already added 30-minutes, and the person who made the appointment for me added another 30-minutes. This is in part why patients spend excessive amounts of time waiting.

Part of the problem is that what scheduled times mean are not consistent. The folks at mammograms, ultrasound, and interventional radiology add the 30-minutes wait time to the online system – your appointment is scheduled 30-minutes later than it says on the system. The folks who do MRI do not add this prep time. I have no idea whether I should be showing up at the appointed time or 30-minutes before the appointed time. If the 30-minutes accounts for parking, tell me that because it doesn't take me 30-minutes to park. Scott drops me off, and parks, which means there are 15-minutes that I don't need added to my pre-appointment time.

Today I asked for a supervisor. Why not? I was waiting anyways; I might as well make use of my time. The supervisor had no idea about this problem and said this was the first time anyone had bothered to complain. There was no awareness that there was an issue. She promised me she would investigate it and inform various people who could fix it. I felt like she was taking my feedback seriously. I felt as though – like they were inspired to better appreciate the patient experience and learn about ways in which to improve their process. I also complained that when I checked in at 8:50 am, almost an hour before my appointment, the receptionist did not tell me how early I was. Had the receptionist told me, I would have gone for a walk, gotten myself a second cup of coffee, or somehow made use of the 55 minutes that I'd be waiting. Instead, I spent the time sitting in the poorly lit waiting room. My general rule is, if you think I'll be waiting more than 15-minutes, then tell me.

The Canadian in me feels guilty for making a stink about it, but the other part of me feels good for asking for the supervisor. My mental state isn't exactly great right now, so I don't always think to ask. You cannot fix a broken system if you don't speak up and tell people it is broken.

One of my biggest pet peeves in this whole cancer treatment process is the amount of wasted time I spend in waiting rooms. It is a huge lost opportunity. How can we make that time more useful, so it isn't just about waiting? I'm open to suggestions.

Social media and patient engagement

I've transitioned in my face-to-face support group from the newbie going through treatment to the experienced breast cancer patient who can answer various questions about chemotherapy.

I use social media to get a sense of the 'lived experience' of a given treatment. When I reach out and ask, I receive experiences from others as well as a boat load of advice. This information is often very useful in helping me better gauge what to expect, but also in helping me ask questions of my healthcare team. This in-turn reminds me of one of the best pieces of advice that I received when I was initially diagnosed: '**decide who you want to trust and trust them** '. I've decided that I trust my oncologist and my surgeon. This means that I can hear advice from various outlets (social media, friends, support groups, etc.) and use that information to pose questions to my care team. From there, I can then remind myself who I trust, and take their advice.

I find myself regularly having to remind myself that I've decided that I trust my oncologist and surgeon – because information from social media can be very disproportionate. What do I mean by disproportionate? When you ask about potential surgery complications, you are going to hear a lot about complications. You won't truly understand how rare some of those complications are – because the people drawn to social media to share their experiences aren't typically people who have had ideal experiences (those people don't feel like they have anything to share) – so a disproportionate amount of what is shared is the exception to the rule rather than the rule itself (at least that is what I believe – I might need to do a study to test this hypothesis). My point is, that my surgeon and oncologist provide an opinion that is grounded in evidence and experience – where social media provides anecdotal evidence. As an engaged patient both are important. I need the social media information to appreciate the lived experience (before it is my experience) and I need the evidence-based advice that my specialists provide. If I had not decided who to trust, I'd have a more difficult time navigating treatment.

For now, the chemo is done

―――――

October 31, 2014

Yesterday was my last scheduled chemotherapy.

Towards the end of treatment, the chemo nurses sang the chemo song. A tear or two did drop from my eyes as they were singing and congratulating me. For the last four treatments, I had been anticipating the moment I finally heard them sing, "Hey now, the chemo is done". The problem is, I don't feel like the chemo is done. Let's start with the fact that this may have been my last infusion, but I still must go through the side effects. I still have a difficult week ahead of me before I start to recover from the chemo. My treatment isn't done. I don't know what the pathology results will show.

Instead of '**Hey** now, the chemo is done', I feel more like '**For** now, the chemo is done'.

From the treatment perspective, focus is now shifting to surgery. Each time I see the surgeon, things change a little. I wanted my breast surgeon to tell me where the incisions were going to be and what I could expect when I wake up from the first surgery. They do the incisions on the first surgery based upon the second surgery, that way they can use the same incisions. Fortunately, Thursday is the day that the plastic surgeons are at the women's centre, so my breast surgeon brought in my plastic surgeon and the two of them discussed and decided where the best place would be for the incisions. Then my breast surgeon drew on my breasts (in ballpoint pen) where the incision will be.

We then talked about pain management. Prior to surgery, I will see nuclear medicine to have an isotope injected to help identify the sentinel node(s) for the sentinel node biopsy. The sentinel nodes are the first lymph nodes outside of the breast. This will involve approximately 4 needles in each breast, each feeling like a bee sting. Then, at the mammography centre, they will use a mammogram machine and place wires that the surgeons use to identify where two of the tumours are. The current plan is to only remove L1 and R1 – one tumour on each breast. Typically, a local anesthetic is used for wire placement. It is still not pleasant with the mammogram machine squeezing, which is extra not fun when you have a port. They don't usually use any anesthesia for the nuclear injections. In most cases, women are only doing this with one breast. My surgeon is connected to the head of pain management in anesthesia (the regional director). Given all the pre-surgery procedures, I've been referred to him to have a para-vertebral nerve block prior to the visit to nuclear medicine for the injections, which in theory means I won't feel anything around the breast area.

All my pre-op appointments are scheduled in the morning. The three hour surgery is scheduled for 1:30 p.m. Then I go to recovery for at least 2 hours, while I wake up. I'm happy to be in the hospital overnight when all the surgery related pain meds will wear off. I'll have ready access to doctors if needed to help with pain management. I'll probably send Scott to the pharmacy to get the pain meds, so we have the drugs in hand when we leave the hospital.

I continue to be impressed with getting little bits of special treatment. I'm a squeaky wheel, in that I booked the extra appointment to see my surgeon because I didn't know where she was placing the incisions and I wanted to know. I'm so glad we had the appointment, as I have a much clearer picture of how things will work on the day of surgery and being a special case for pain management will also mean my personal experience will be a little less painful.

Familiar fatigue

November 4, 2014

This morning, I found myself struggling to get moving. Then it occurred to me, I'm feeling fatigued. I haven't felt this type of fatigue since AC chemo. I'm encouraged by the fatigue. During AC chemo, I was able to combat the worst of the fatigue with exercise.

The challenge I have now is exercising with neuropathy. This whole neuropathy experience is nothing like I expected. I didn't expect neuropathy to come with pain, as it was always described as 'pins-and-needles'. Now I'm finding that neuropathy is coming with tense muscles. When I use my numb feet or hands, my calves and forearms get really tense.

Not being able to drive makes self-care more difficult. Yes, that is a bit of an excuse, but only a bit. I could always take the train, taxis, or ask someone for a ride. I have been doing that a little more often than I'd like. It is a barrier to getting out. There is a loss of freedom that happens when you cannot get in the car and go. I hope that my inability to drive is temporary and that, as the effects of Paclitaxel fade, my ability to drive returns. For now, I'll start with walking. If I can walk without visual cognition issues, then I can consider a short drive, avoiding highways. Hopefully by the end of the week I'll be back behind the wheel.

The good news is the fatigue is familiar. It is something that I know I can manage. I have a strategy to deal with it.

What do you do?

November 7, 2014

What do you do? Such a simple question, and yet one that is crazy difficult to answer right now.

I consider exercise and writing my full-time job. What I do right now is write, exercise, and try to gather strength for surgery.

In the cancer community, the question isn't asked that often. When it is, there is an understanding that right now I'm "in treatment". What I do is treatment. But when I'm with a new group of people at church or another social event, the question is immensely difficult and rather awkward. Do I say that I'm in treatment for cancer?

I was doing a PhD, but right now, I'm on leave. I was a part-time professor. Although I still use that occasionally, it is somewhat dishonest – I'm part of the part-time professors' union. You are a member for 2 years after you teach a class. I'm not teaching right now, and likely won't be teaching anytime soon. I am, however, doing some research as a part-time professor.

I'm also a consultant. I produce eBooks for the iBooks Store. When I'm not in active treatment, I'd like to do more of this. I like helping people self-publish.

The question wasn't always that easy to answer before cancer, but I could say, "I'm working on a PhD", or I'm a freelance eBook Producer (in the US the term freelance is used, in Canada it is more common to use the term consultant) – both of which were conversation starters. The cancer answer is often more of a conversation killer.

For now, what I do is exercise and write. One step at a time.

Chemo recall

November 9, 2014

I had hoped that with each day past my regular infusion day, my side effects would start to get better. Unfortunately, some of them are getting worse. It is as if my body remembers that on this day you get a new dose of chemo, so the cumulative effects should continue to get worse. Now, in addition to stopping the chemo, I'm also not taking any steroids (one of the chemo pre-meds). So, I'm not getting the thing that boosted me up each week.

Today I'm feeling nerve pain, which is causing my muscles (mostly in my calves and forearms) to go tense. My feet are totally numb. My joints are weak. It is rather frustrating, as I want to be feeling better, feeling stronger, feeling ready for an activity filled vacation in Hawaii. I continue to remind myself that recovery will take time, one day at a time.

Smoothies, turtles, and going topless

November 14, 2014

We have fallen into a bit of a morning routine here on Maui. Get up and make a coffee and breakfast smoothies, watch the turtles playing in the surf from the lanai (patio) of our condo, then head out for a morning snorkel. The snorkelling itself hasn't been as good as it was back in February – perhaps I'm remembering wrong, but I recall seeing more fish when I was here back in February.

While snorkelling, I found myself struggling with the logistics of how to go topless. If you recall, the entire purpose of this trip was to go snorkelling topless with the turtles. I knew I wanted to do it but couldn't figure out how to manage it. There aren't that many places to discretely enter / exit the water without a top on. Fortunately, Nicky figured it out – it was just a matter of wearing a one-piece bathing suit, and slipping down the straps. With this technique, I can easily go topless without having to worry about losing any articles of clothing, and I can easily put my top back on before making my way back to shore.

With the logistics figured out, I give it a try. It is wonderful. There is a whole new sense of freedom when you swim topless.

Unfortunately, there were no turtles where we were snorkelling. They all seem to be hanging out just outside of our condo.

On the neuropathy front, things aren't going so well. I hoped that as time progressed the neuropathy would get better. Honestly, I had hoped that within a week of ending chemo most of the neuropathy would have gone away! My expectations of recovery were overly ambitious to say the least. My ankles are swollen, and my calves and forearms are all knotted up. Fortunately, this does not seem to negatively impact my ability to snorkel; however, it does impact my ability to walk. For now, I'm getting my exercise snorkelling in the morning and napping in the afternoon. We'll see how things over the weekend.

A photo shoot and getting ready for surgery

November 18, 2014

Never in my life did I imagine that I'd be posing naked in a photo studio just north of Berkeley, California! Cancer has certainly meant I've found myself doing a lot of those 'never' things.

At a cancer survivor conference that I attended, there was an exhibit of photos on each table. The photos were elegant pictures that celebrated women's breasts. The photos really spoke to me, so I emailed the photographer about a possible session. Since I was unable to drive or get a ride, I ended up booking for today – the only possible time to take the photos before surgery. It was rather fortunate that her schedule and my schedule aligned. I was much more nervous about my ability to drive than about having photos taken. It is the first time I've driven on my own up through Oakland to Berkeley. I was rather intimidated to drive on that highway, which is often full of traffic. Fortunately, it turned out to not be so bad. I found myself in a photo studio just north of Berkeley, posing for an elegant set of photos that celebrate my breasts. I really enjoyed the process and am looking forward to seeing the photos. When I get them, I'll share a few of the 'general public friendly' photos here. I recommend the session for anyone who wants to capture their pre-surgery selves.

I need to get back to my pre-surgery preparations: getting some food ready for when I get home. I need to shower before trying to get a little bit of sleep. I will shower again in the morning before driving up to the university hospital for a 6 a.m. start. Surgery isn't until 1:40 pm, but there are several pre-surgery procedures. Specifically, injection of some nuclear isotope into each breast that helps to identify the sentinel node, and the insertion of wires to guide the surgeon to the exact location of each of the tumours, neither of which sounds at all like fun.

One of my concerns with surgery is that I'm highly sensitive to adhesives. Even steri-strips cause skin blisters. If any tape or adhesive based dressing is used, it will blister within a few hours – making me very uncomfortable but also hindering my body's ability to heal. Fortunately, they don't need to use adhesives, they just need to be reminded to not use them. Rather than adhesives, they use special surgical glue to close the incision. My husband came up with the idea of adding a note in permanent marker on my belly, just under my breasts. I'll have him write 'no tape' as a reminder to not put anything sticky on my skin.

An update from the hospital

———

November 20, 2014

I told Scott before surgery that the one piece of information I wanted when I woke up was the status of the sentinel node biopsy. I was right. Scott tells me that I asked at least five times while in the recovery room and was happy each time he told me they were clear. The surgeon just came into my hotel hospital room to tell me that "the preliminary results are clear but that they are preliminary results". It is very good news, but it is to be taken with a caution as they haven't done the more detailed pathology. The preliminary results are 90% accurate. I'm completely relieved. The sentinel nodes are typically the first place that breast cancer spreads. If my nodes come back from pathology as clear, then my cancer was caught at Stage 2.

After a longer visit with the Surgical Fellow, I got more details. They took 2 or 3 nodes from each side – a little more on the left. They like to take at least 2 for pathology. She emphasized that there was a very small risk of lymphedema (swelling of the arms due to a blockage in the lymph drainage system). The bigger concern over the next week was to avoid things that might tear incisions or injure the surgery sites.

We had an OK night's sleep. They gave us a private room, so Scott was able to stay the night. This turned out to be very useful, as several times I benefitted from having a patient advocate (things like helping when I needed to use the toilet). He was here for most of the doctor and nurse visits.

In surgery, they put these gentle massage cuffs that are sort of like blood pressure cuffs but with less air. It is done to avoid blood clots but has also helped with the tight knotted calves that are a result of neuropathy and swollen ankles.

The Stanford hospital uses a room service model for food, which is impressive. The menu is quite good, and so far, the food has been good. The food is locally sourced where possible, and there are organic options. There are even organic options for those on a liquid diet. This is one area where I think it makes a huge difference in patient wellness. The food has been good enough that we decided to check out after lunch rather than before. That way I'll go home well drugged and with a full belly.

Ya No!

―――

November 23, 2014

Ya, no ... That is pretty much what I thought when the resident on call suggested a catheter with a pee bag attached to my leg for the next week or so.

I don't think she really heard me right. I said I was having difficulty urinating, but I am still doing it! There is still pee coming out of me ... perhaps not as much as there should be.

Over the phone, she diagnosed me with post-operative urinary retention, which is the most common side effect of anesthesia, according to a quick Google search. I was hoping for some anti-spasm drugs (like you sometimes get for a urinary tract infection), to allow my body to relax when I try to pee, but no such luck. The problem is that the involuntary muscles aren't working properly. The resident explained that my bladder is still "asleep" — it has not yet woken up from the anesthesia.

Sensing my non-compliance, she asked if I was okay with the plan. I said, "No, how about we watch and wait? — because I am passing some urine, I'm not completely blocked — it is just taking time and not flowing properly". I don't completely trust the resident's opinion and want to hear it from someone with more experience. I have an appointment with my surgeon (whom I trust) tomorrow at 10 a.m. The resident and I negotiated a plan. I will watch and wait, but if I have a window of six to eight hours where I don't pass any urine or if I feel my bladder is full or distended, then I'm to go to an urgent care centre and ask for a catheter and leg bag. I must give the resident credit for detecting, by the sound of my voice, that I had no intention of just going in and getting the catheter and bag. We spent a few minutes discussing the watch and wait option, so I know what signs mean I need to go and get it dealt with.

Now that I've had a little more time to process the idea, I can deal with it. If my surgeon says I need it, I will get it tomorrow and deal with it while travelling (oh joy). The resident said that it would stay in for a week, and then they would do some test to see if my bladder was working properly (voiding) so that it could be removed.

On the pain front, I've started to wean off the pain meds. I'm on a lower dose, less frequently, and so far, it is working out. I caught myself last night unconsciously doing my normal inspection of my breasts, and I accidentally squeezed one of them a little. Hurt like ...

... won't be doing that again anytime too soon!

A surgeon who understands

———

November 24, 2014

Mostly today's visit was just a checkup before flying to Canada on Wednesday. I wanted to make sure everything was healing as expected. It is. My surgeon took a bunch of pictures of her handiwork for both my file and for research. All is well.

The pathology isn't in yet, but the preliminary results of the nodes are negative. In addition, the preliminary results of the tissue under the nipples are also negative. This is good news. If there is any cancer in the tissue under the nipples, then the nipples will be removed when I have the mastectomy on December 17. If the tissue under the nipples remains negative, then the goal will be to keep the nipples as part of the surgery December 17 (bilateral mastectomy with immediate deep inferior epigastric perforators flap reconstruction, known as DIEP flap reconstruction). We will get a full pathology report on December 4.

When we discussed my bladder issues, my surgeon commented that maybe it is because she is an older doctor, but she finds that sometimes she needs to remind residents to consider the patient perspective before making recommendations. This was a classic and interesting example — before suggesting a catheter and pee bag for a week, think about the patient impact. My surgeon agreed with the watch and wait approach given my upcoming trip, and if it is still a problem when I get back, she can refer me to urology for a consult. She would rather give me a referral to a specialist than put me through the unnecessary discomfort of a week with a catheter and pee bag. It really confirmed that I had chosen the right surgeon — one that looks at me as a person, and my entire well-being, not just my symptoms.

Flyin'

———

November 26, 2014

Today will be my first post-surgery flight. It has only been a week since surgery. In the surgery, I had a sentinel lymph node dissection (SLND) on both sides (bilateral). If I were to listen to the various breast cancer support group sites, I should be flying with compression sleeves on both arms, because the removal of lymph nodes means I'm at increased risk for lymphedema. If you listen to this rhetoric, you might think that my arms will immediately swell upon entering the airplane. Fortunately, there are cases of lymphedema, but they are not as prevalent as the various patient communities would make you think.

One of my challenges is that the precautionary advice regarding things to avoid in the affected arm (e.g. needles, blood pressure) can usually be done in the unaffected arm. I don't have an unaffected arm, so, I need to analyze the risks more deeply. Is it a risk or an unnecessary precaution? Good question!

Doing what I can to improve the experience for others

December 1, 2014

On Wednesday, November 19th I was wheeled around to various departments as part of my pre-surgery preparation. I was seen by mammography, where they placed three wires in my breasts. These wires were guides for the surgeons – to show them where each of my tumours were.

When I returned from my Thanksgiving trip to Canada, I discovered that I'd received three letters in the mail, each stating that the mammogram that I had on November 19th was "normal". I had heard about this happening. Often, organizations send out annual mammogram reminders to women who have had double-mastectomies (you don't do mammograms when you don't have any natural breast tissue).

Rather than dismissing the letters – I sent along an email to the supervisor I had chatted with back when we had issues with wait times in mammography. Since the supervisor gave me her card, I decided to use it.

Now the supervisor knows that the automated system is sending out these letters at times when it is inappropriate. She knows that the system is broken and can now report it to someone who can fix it. Before my email, she was completely unaware this was happening.

As an engaged patient part of my responsibility is to report broken systems. If I tell someone who can then report the problem to someone who can fix it, then I'm doing my part to help improve the systems for everyone that follows.

I am hoping that women who are undergoing treatment for breast cancer no longer get reports of "normal" mammograms for procedures to help remove the cancer. Let's save the "normal" results for post treatment when we can celebrate them!

Swollen ankles and crazy nails

December 3, 2014

I've been experiencing stiffness in my ankles for over a month now. I blamed neuropathy on the stiffness. I wasn't using my ankles properly while walking, causing my calves to get nasty knots in them. In Canada, using Voltaren gel provided a significant improvement in mobility in my ankles.

Although I thought my ankles were swollen before, something happened on Monday afternoon, and they became a different kind of swollen. I kind of feel like the Pillsbury Dough Boy ... the rest of me isn't swollen, other than my breasts – which still have some post-surgery swelling), but these ankles are a little crazy (they are less swollen first thing in the morning), see Image 17. When you add neuropathy on top of swollen, things feel rather unusual.

Today I'm waiting for a call from the doctor's office. My oncologist called last night – and has ordered a Doppler test for some time today to see how the blood is flowing in my legs.

You'll notice from the picture that my big toes are discoloured. I'm expecting to lose them sometime soon, but I've never lost a nail before, so I have no idea how the process works. I'm going to see a nail specialist on Thursday to ensure there is no infection. The discolouration and nail loss are side effects of the Paclitaxel chemo. My fingernails are also funky colours, but the damaged nail seems to be growing out normally.

Pathology – What it says

December 6, 2014

On Thursday I received the first surgical pathology report. I'll get another at the end of the month after my bilateral mastectomy. This one reported on nine tissue samples that were taken on my November 19th surgery.

First and foremost, my nodes remain "negative for carcinoma". In addition, the sub-nipple biopsy also indicates negative for carcinoma. That means, that my upcoming surgery on December 17th will be a nipple sparing bilateral mastectomy with immediate flap reconstruction. The surgeons will do what they can to keep my nipples (yay). It may not seem like much to someone who isn't going through this process, but the whole idea of looking down after surgery and seeing yourself has a huge psychological impact. As much as I may not feel that I 'care' about my nipples, I know that if they were gone, I would really feel it. Since the technique is rather specialized, I'm also contributing to the education of residents and fellows during the process. For me, that gives some meaning to this horrible experience. It makes it important.

The next part of the pathology talks about the three lumpectomies. I had three known tumours based upon the initial pre-chemo MRI. L1 was the largest mass at 2.4cm x 2.3cm x 3.0cm. L2 was a small mass only found on MRI at 1.0cm x .9cm x .8cm. R1 was a mass 2.7 cm x 2.1 cm x 2.0 cm. The earlier biopsies showed DCIS in the left breast. It is not uncommon to see DCIS (pre-cancerous cells) when there is IDC. In addition, chemotherapy doesn't target DCIS.

L1 – This was the biggest success. What was left in the area was scar tissue with a single .2cm cancerous mass. In addition, there was DCIS close to the margin (in essence, if I had been only doing a lumpectomy, this would be said as not having clean margins therefore additional surgery is required. But in my case, it doesn't matter because they are going to remove all the breast tissue on the next surgery).

L2 – This showed only normal tissue. **My guess** here is that they got the wrong spot because the marker was out of place. We will find out more about this in the mastectomy pathology.

R1 – This showed the part that worries me the most. This showed a mass of 2.1 cm x 1.6 cm of IDC and additional DCIS. 10% of the invasive mass was DCIS. Here the margins were not at all clear with additional invasion at the margins. What concerns me most is that the chemo had little effect on this mass. It is a little smaller (so at least it isn't bigger), but not significantly so.

The pathology included staging for my cancer:

- Left: ypT1a ypN0 (post neo-adjuvant chemotherapy, stage 1A no lymph nodes)
- Right: ypT2 ypN0 (post neo-adjuvant chemotherapy, stage 2 no lymph nodes)

In summary, the left breast shows definite signs that the chemo worked, where on the right the treatment effect is listed as "indeterminate".

Pathology – What it means

December 7, 2014

I've gotten pretty good at interpreting what the pathology reports say, but I'm not great at what it means.

Just before my oncologist walked into the room I said to Scott, "What I'm afraid of is that he will recommend more chemotherapy".

My oncologist said that he would be presenting my case at the case conference the next day, where all the cancer specialists get together and collectively try to figure out the best course of action. The question was, do I need more chemotherapy after surgery, and if so, what chemotherapy?

I didn't think to ask my oncologist why he thought I might need more chemo – but I'm guessing it is because of the R1 results. This is the first time my oncologist mentioned the bilateral nature of my cancer and how bilateral cancer is rare – which is in part why they don't have a clear path for treatment. In addition, they have only been doing neo-adjuvant chemotherapy for 15-years – so again, longer term outcomes are not completely clear. I'm pretty sure that if we were only dealing with L1, the idea of more chemo would not have been suggested.

This question determines whether my port will be removed on my upcoming surgery on December 17th. If more chemotherapy is needed, then the port stays, otherwise it can be removed (making the breast and plastic surgeons' jobs easier).

Fortunately, on Friday afternoon I got word that, "Case conference discussed your case. No more chemo indicated; we will take out your port at the time of surgery. You will be recommended to take 5 years of Tamoxifen after surgery. No more chemo!" I broke down in tears after reading this.

Yay on the *no more chemo*. I'm cautiously optimistic that the recommendation will remain the same after my next surgery when the full breast pathology is available, but I'm still nervous about the R1 result – the chemo didn't really work on that tumour, does it mean that I'm destined for recurrence? Or will the surgery be enough to kick this cancer?

Looking back at the data about complete pathological response in neo-adjuvant chemo, the left breast response is good – it was close to a complete pathological response and may very well have been one had I completed the three additional doses of Paclitaxel. That looks good. That fact that I did not have a clear indication of response in the right breast is a predictor of absolutely nothing (since the tumour wasn't as big nor growing as fast – complete pathological response isn't an indicator of prognosis). That is, it in no way predicts whether my cancer will metastasize. It is pretty much a roll of the dice ... only time will tell.

New energy means renewed ability to get stressed

December 12, 2014

My energy returns, and I'm stuck with the daunting task of prioritizing all the things on my to-do list – all those things that I've been avoiding or just plain not doing because I could not concentrate or did not have the energy. Now I'm so crazy overwhelmed with a to do list a mile long, that all I want to do is turn off my computer, pick up my laptop and watch TV ... oh the vicious cycle.

As my brain starts working again, the scope of this next surgery starts to dawn on me. Each time I get in the shower, I ask myself – am I making the right decision? What if I changed my mind and opted for breast conserving surgery (lumpectomy) ... then I remember, first off, that there is still cancer in my breasts after the last surgery (that sneaky little L2 that is difficult to find on mammograms), my margins were not clear which means they would need more surgery to get a clean margin around the cancer. Then if they did manage to get all the invasive stuff out, my breasts also have DCIS which is harder to find, and then I would need radiation on both sides, and when all that was done, I'd need to return every 6-months for a mammogram or MRI to ensure that the cancer hasn't returned. I'm sure that if I asked my doctors, they would all say that the bilateral mastectomy is the right decision to treat my cancer.

About 10 days after surgery, I'll get another pathology report – this time on all the breast tissue that is removed during the mastectomy. It will be this report that will help to elucidate the true extent of the cancer – or at least the post-chemotherapy result.

What frustrates me is that I know that some of the cancer reacted well to the chemo regime I was on, and some of it did not.

My renewed sense of energy means that I'm getting stressed out all over again. I need to try to re-focus my energy on positive things – on moving forward. If the weather clears tomorrow, I shall focus on going for a nice walk. Then I need to start preparing for surgery Wednesday and my in-laws arriving Friday. Now I just need to find a little focus.

Getting organized at home

———

December 23, 2014

Over the next few days, I'll try and get caught up on reporting about my hospital experience. It was a mixed experience, certainly not all positive, but I had some terrific nurses and nurse assistants, and a pretty terrific husband caregiver too – which made it go much better than it otherwise would have.

When we got home, one of the biggest challenges was figuring out all the medications and a schedule that allows us to create an efficient process. I can now better appreciate why it felt like the nurses were giving me various pills on an almost hourly basis. I'm at 17 different meds, with 11 different dose times. The goal in setting up a schedule was to optimize pain medications and reduce the number of times in the day I'm taking drugs, while still respecting various drug interactions. This isn't something that is easily done by the pharmacy, as the pharmacy doesn't deal with all the over-the-counter meds that are also prescribed (e.g. I'm prescribed certain vitamins which aren't provided by the pharmacy).

After several hours and a phone call to the hospital, he was able to prioritize drug interactions. It was possible to meet some of the requirements, just not all of them. He created a spreadsheet of when to take which meds. It would have been a lot more useful if the hospital had printed out my medication schedule for the last 48-hours I was in the hospital. That would have given Scott something to work with. I cannot imagine how the average person could even begin to manage this.

Initially we had not included my asthma inhalers in the medications to take at home. In the hospital, a separate respiratory tech would visit me twice a day, to give me one of my asthma inhalers. The one they gave me was different than what I normally take. The hospital often makes substitutes to align with their systems and availability. Since it wasn't what I normally took, I didn't think about it when I got home. Then after dinner, I suddenly had an asthma attack.

I had Scott and my in-laws rushing around the house trying to find inhalers and pillows and whatever to try to reduce the pain induced with the sudden onset of coughing and wheezing. It was NOT fun. I then realized why they were proactively giving me an inhaler while in hospital. Now we have added proactive inhalers to my list of meds.

So far, so good.

Initial impressions

December 25, 2014

The first time I looked down at my new breasts, the day after surgery as the dressings were being changed, my first thought was that they were a little smaller than I expected. I had told my plastic surgeon that I'd be happy with about a 20% reduction in size, but somehow, I had not internalized what that would be like. Also, since the cancer began growing, my breasts were not 'normal'. Over the last 6-months they have been continually changing. I no longer know what 'normal' would be. What I can say is that when I look down, I see breasts. With each day, my breasts seem to be a different size, swelling and then receding, like the river behind the condo. It may be a month or two before they stabilize into a 'size'.

My new breasts (noobs), look a lot like my old breasts. This is because the replaced parts are all under the skin. The skin is my original breast skin. It is still very difficult to tell how the nipples will turn out. They were initially saved during the surgery, but it isn't completely clear yet if the blood flow will re-establish correctly and what things will look like when the wounds heal.

What came as a bit of a surprise was that when I look down between my breasts, I now see a flat belly. I'm really impressed at how well that turned out.

The end of active treatment

———

December 29, 2014

Emotions flood over me in waves. Whenever I think about it, I cannot stop crying. It has been a roller coaster of a journey, and it is now officially over!

What do I mean? As of Dec 17th, I'm cancer free. The double mastectomy removed the last bits of cancer from my breasts. The pathology showed a .7cm mass in my left breast – the ever-elusive L2 that wasn't found in the first surgery. Other than that, everything else was clear, including the lymph nodes within the breasts. My surgeon said she saw no reason for radiation – and to follow up in a month to see how the incisions are healing.

My oncologist said that he was surprised that all my nodes were clear. The prognosis is much better given that the cancer never spread beyond the breast tissue. Now that I don't have any breast tissue left, the only places for non-metastatic spread are against the chest wall and on the skin and incisions.

Today marks the end of active treatment. My tears are of relief ... it is finally over.

The next step is a pill called Tamoxifen (prescription has been sent to my pharmacy), which is taken once a day for 10 years (or until my body goes into menopause – at which time it is switched over to an Aromatase Inhibitor). This pill suppresses my body's ability to create estrogen, the primary thing that fed my cancer. I am to start Tamoxifen once I am a little more healed from the surgery. This allows them to know what is causing what symptoms. The surgery itself was major. My body needs a few more weeks to heal.

Now I need to wean myself off the pain meds so that I can enjoy a good glass of wine to celebrate the new year – free of cancer – starting over.

Recovery is still a long road. My hematocrit tanked again (lower than ever), which means my red blood cells are low. I find myself easily out of breath while walking or climbing a single flight of stairs. My incisions are healing well. I still have a couple of drains which I'll probably have until next Monday as they are still producing a fair amount of fluid. For the next week, we shall take one step at a time, trying to increase my walking distance and awaiting the day when I can get back on the bike.

An engaged patient needs an engaged caregiver

———

December 31, 2014

It was never clearer than when I was in the hospital, that I needed my husband, and I needed him to be just as engaged in my care as I was (or perhaps even more so). There were several times when things were not quite right, but I was not in any shape to explain what was wrong. I was too drugged up to provide a true picture of how I was feeling or what my concerns were. That was when my husband stepped in and explained things. He listened intently when the doctors were giving instructions, and often found that he needed to clarify things for the nurses. I had some awesome nurses, but they were not there when the doctor explained how to dress the wounds. My husband was. He was the one person who ensured that I had continuity in my care.

Coming home from the hospital posed its own challenges. We were unable to get an electric recliner but had several wedge pillows. With the help of the physical therapist at the hospital I was able to get into and out of bed on my own. However, I wasn't able to stack the necessary pillows under my knees and feet. To reduce ankle swelling I need to sleep with my feet elevated, so every time I get out of bed in the night, I need help getting set back up so that I can sleep. I was also very lucky that our patio rocking chairs happened to be just the right height and have just the right resistance, such that I had a comfortable place to sit when I wasn't sleeping.

At home, my husband plays the role of nurse. I have several incisions that require dressing changes once or twice per day. Because we both like efficient processes, we have figured out efficient ways to manage these changes. My hubby strips and empties drains the first thing in the morning, then removes all dressings so that I can shower. After I'm all dried off, pictures are taken, then all wounds are dressed for the day. The process takes over an hour but seems to be the most efficient time for changing dressing as I'm already undressed and clean.

Then there are all the pills. I don't have the mental capacity (especially with the pain meds) to figure out when to take which pills. Managing this has been no small task (we reduced a few when we saw the doctors on Monday and hope a few more go away next week).

I must emphasize that there is no way I could be an engaged patient without the help of my husband – who is a very engaged caregiver.

Today, I say thank-you to my loving husband for all his support through this ordeal, and I wish him a very happy birthday.

A small cup of coffee

January 2, 2015

Recovery is slow. Although I was happy to announce the end of active treatment, I still need to recover from that treatment.

I was lucky in that I only had two surgeries. Many women go through this process with a lot more surgeries that are a lot further spread out and are in treatment for 2-3 years. The nipple sparing mastectomy saved me at least one surgery (or tattoo) – one to recreate nipples. Doing the reconstruction at the same time as the double mastectomy also saved me surgeries. The combined surgery is not an option for many women.

I will likely have one more surgery, but there will be no rush. There will be no worries of cancer growing or spreading. The surgery can be scheduled after I've gained my strength – at a time when I feel strong going into it.

With each day I make a few more steps towards recovery. Today was a 3.2 km walk – just shy of 5000 steps. We will do a second walk over to Safeway later today.

I've also started to reduce my pain meds, so that I can eventually enjoy a glass of wine with dinner. Alas, healing takes time. Pain needs to remain managed, otherwise the healing process will go slower. Rushing to reduce the pain meds will cause more trouble than slowly weaning off them.

On the good news, I got clearance from my plastic surgery nurse to have a small cup of coffee. I enjoyed a very nice cup of Kauai coffee that we bought when we were in Hawaii in November. I stopped all caffeine (coffee and chocolate) a week and a half before surgery. Since the surgery involved microscopically connecting blood vessels, I needed to stop eating/drinking anything that made those vessels smaller. Now that I'm two weeks out from surgery and healing nicely, I've received clearance for a little coffee. This goes a long way to reducing the pain meds, as caffeine makes some of the pain meds more effective. My one small cup of coffee (and perhaps a little regular chocolate) will go a long way to helping me heal.

I am thankful for all the walking and biking I did before surgery. When I took my first steps, my legs were strong. It made a huge difference to how quickly I was able to move, and how quickly I've been able to walk.

Today I am thankful for my small cup of coffee.

Ups and Downs

January 5, 2015

Healing is full of ups and downs. One day you are doing well, and then the next, not so much.

Saturday, I really overdid it. I walked over 5km, then went to two support groups which meant I was sitting for four hours.

To top that off, I tried to taper off my overnight pain meds.

It didn't work out so well. We had planned on being up early on Sunday in preparation for Scott going back to work Monday. We need to ensure routines are in place so that I've showered and had all my dressings changed before he goes to work. Of course, that didn't happen. I didn't sleep well (less pain meds after a long day), so we didn't get up early, and I took it easy most of Sunday.

On a Facebook group, someone posted this video that graphically shows a procedure pretty like what I had; although, I'm pretty sure that my plastic surgeon didn't cut out a piece of my rib, but we'll check that today. I made it through about 1/2 the video before stopping. It was just too much but did help explain why I'm feeling pain inside where my belly button is. It helps to appreciate just how involved this surgery is, and why it might take a while to deal with the pain of healing.

Today, I'm looking forward to hearing what the plastic surgeon says. It was comforting to see my surgeon daily or every other day in the hospital. Yet it is much harder to go for a week without seeing a surgeon to ensure the wounds are healing. Looking at the photos, it looks like my incisions are healing nicely.

Healing on the outside doesn't reflect how well I'm healing on the inside. My incisions may not hurt but I feel a general pain on the inside, like my insides have been turned upside down and backwards and are still settling into their new locations. The pain is mostly on the inside, which makes it difficult to describe.

But with each day, I'm getting stronger, feeling more energy (except Sunday). As long as I don't overdo, then I shall be fine. Crossing my fingers, I get these drains out soon and ride the trike on the weekend.

And then there was one

———

January 13, 2015

I was really hoping to have both my drains pulled today, but neither had output low enough to warrant being pulled (close but not quite). I wonder if it had more to do with my mental health than anything else. They did remove one of the remaining abdominal drains. Now I wait another week with one drain. Better one than two, but I really wanted to see both go. Fortunately, the drain removal itself felt like nothing. I didn't notice it at all. It will be interesting to see if the output of the remaining drain increases because it is now the only abdominal drain.

Once I have two days in a row with low enough output then I can call, and they will pull the final drain. I also have an appointment with my plastic surgeon on Thursday next week, so the final drain might end up going then. I might hold the record for the longest drains, as of tomorrow it will be 4 weeks (ugh).

I'm also feeling achy, and my joints are really sore. I didn't walk again today in part because my left foot hurt too much, causing me to limp. It was better that I do not walk and hope that the foot is feeling better tomorrow. The joints seem stiffer today and the walking makes the joints feel better. I'm looking forward to being able to do other forms of exercise and plan on being on a bike one week after the drains come out.

I've signed up for a cancer exercise program at the local Y that starts January 28. I'm hoping that by then I don't have drains and I'm mostly off the pain meds. The program is a light workout, but also gives me full access to the Y. I can take any of their classes (Zumba and cardio belly dance look interesting to me – might be a while before I'm ready for either of those), including the ones in the pool. Once my incisions have healed, I'll be able to swim again, which will be nice on my sore joints. It will feel very weird and interesting to be in the water and not have feeling on parts of my breasts and stomach. Perhaps this will be similar to how I felt swimming with neuropathy when I couldn't feel parts of my skin in my legs and feet but could feel temperature, just not the sensation of the water.

It will also be interesting to see how I feel about changing and showering at the gym. My body has a lot of new scars. I'm not particularly vain, so I'd like to think that I'd be OK with just changing and not worrying. If someone stares, I can always say, "This is what breast cancer looks like." But really, that is their problem, not mine.

Celebrating my boob job

January 18, 2015

Several women in the breast cancer blogosphere have commented on how inappropriate it is to say to someone with breast cancer that "at least you get a free boob job" or any variant thereof. I agree. If you have never had breast cancer, you do not understand how difficult reconstruction is – especially after your body has gone through chemotherapy and/or radiation treatments, which make reconstruction that much more difficult. It is certainly not a route that most of us would have chosen to go through. On top of that, reconstruction is also a difficult personal choice – to choose the physical pain of the surgery over the emotional well-being and struggle with body image.

As someone who is still recovering, but recently (Dec 17) had a double-nipple-sparing-mastectomy with immediate DIEP Flap reconstruction (a 10-hour surgery), I have the right to celebrate my new breasts (noobs). I am one of the luckier ones – I didn't need radiation as part of my cancer treatment. I did neo-adjuvant chemotherapy, which meant that my reconstruction did not need to be delayed. I got through the worst of the surgeries in two surgeries. I'll have a third to clean things up once the current one has fully healed. Instead of years of reconstruction, I have a reasonable hope of being done with surgery before the end of 2015. The reconstruction surgery wasn't 100% successful, in that I did lose some skin in the process. My nipples aren't what they used to be, but they are still all mine and I won't need to go through the process of nipple reconstruction. My noobs are perky. Now that four weeks have passed, I'm allowed to set them free. I can go without a bra. I tried one of my favourite shirts on, one that I always needed a bra to wear, and I'm quite happy with how it looks. It will look even better when I'm not wearing the abdominal binder. I need to wear the binder for another 4-weeks. It almost feels like my original Buddha belly but even as the picture shows, I do have a slimmer profile (and I'm still a bit swollen overall from the surgery). I'm sure the post-cancer me will look 'healthier' and slimmer than the pre-cancer me – which is rather ironic.

This brings us to another cancer language 'trap' as Nancy Stordahl calls them (Stordahl, 2015). That of cancer being a 'gift'. Honestly, I would rather go back to the pre-cancer me – the lumpy chubby me. The one that was strong and growing stronger each day as I enjoyed regular 30+km bike rides. I may grow through this experience – as we grow through all of life's experiences, but this last eight months has been anything but a gift.

As I struggle through the aches and pains of recovery, I will celebrate how I look even when I'm not yet feeling great. Feel free to tell me, 'You look great' ... but don't ever use the term 'free boob job' unless you, too, have experienced a breast cancer reconstruction, in which case, we can share that 'insider' experience.

The war metaphor

———

January 19, 2015

As much as I hate war, I must admit that the war metaphor for cancer is working for me right now.

There are many bloggers who talk about what is wrong with the war metaphor (fighting cancer, cancer as a battle, etc.) and how that metaphor is problematic when someone doesn't survive or when they are diagnosed metastatic and winning is not achievable. I get the problems with cancer and the war metaphor.

And yet, it is so working for me in this moment. Over the last week and a half, I have been dealing with horrible joint pain—joint pain that sometimes makes it difficult to get out of bed, get out of a chair, get on and off the toilet. Joint pain that is leading to depression, as I am having difficulty seeing the light at the end of the tunnel right now. Don't worry, I am getting help and going for walks, which is the only method of exercise I'm allowed to do.

When I'm walking, struggling to put one step in front of the other, and my iPod shuffles to "The Warrior" by Scandal I am energized. I am reminded that **I CAN DO THIS** because **I AM A WARRIOR**. I so need that right now. For me, in this moment, the war metaphor is working.

See-saw days

January 20, 2015

I think the hardest part of surgical recovery are the see-saw days. What I mean by that is the constant change between days where you are seeing significant improvements and days where you are feeling significantly worse. Day-after-day the ups-and-downs become more and more challenging.

Mentally, I'm feeling better. Physically, not so much. Today's physical struggles are related to sleeping without the wedge pillow last night. I really wanted to sleep on my side – which I did successfully. The problem was that when I was too hot, I didn't have the strength to remove the blankets. When I was too cold, same thing, no strength. For the later part of my night's sleep, I slept on my back without the wedge and was too flat. I dreamed that I was carrying groceries and then jumped into a swimming pool and then I was unable to get myself out. It was just me and the side of the pool, but the water level was too low. There was no way I could get out. It was 1.5 feet from the water level to the edge of pool. Then suddenly it was only a few inches from the water level to the edge, and then I woke up with abdominal pain. My abdomen is not yet ready for the flatness of the bed. I took some pain meds, put the wedge pillow back on the bed, and promptly fell into a silent, dream free sleep for a couple more hours (thank-you pain meds).

We will wait a week or two more before we try that experiment again. It means physically today is going to be rough. I need to keep reminding myself, it is OK, to up the pain meds today. After a difficult night, I need the extra help. Reducing pain meds should happen on good days, not bad ones.

Mentally, I'm feeling stronger and coping better with the joint pain. I'm typing and thinking more. I may even start to do some more planning. I'm thinking about academic stuff again, and potential pathways for the future.

Selfies

―――

January 23, 2015

While walking today I found myself reflecting on why I no longer take selfies when I walk. Early on, and throughout chemotherapy, I always took a selfie of me smiling while I walked along the trail. I don't do that anymore.

One reason is that I'm in theory finished with treatment. Although my body aches, I am done with cancer. I started taking selfies because I wanted there to be lots of pictures of me smiling. If I didn't make it, there would be lots of happy memories for my funeral. Sounds morbid, but that, in part was what I was thinking. I also wanted to show my family who live on the other side of the continent, that I was doing OK. My smile was the one thing you saw in every picture – to show that I'm doing just fine.

I am still walking, and this weekend I will start biking again. My plastic surgeon did caution me, that I'm still healing. She was clear, until eight weeks have passed, I'm healing and I'm not to overdo it. I don't want to overdo it; I just want to do it. Walking is painful. I'm slow, but my feet also hurt. The neuropathy pain gets worse the more I walk, making it is challenging, but since it is the only exercise I can do, I do it almost every day. I'm so looking forward to adding biking into the mix. Crossing my fingers, it all works out.

Everything yet nothing is cancer

January 26, 2015

At this stage, every ache causes me to question, then dismiss cancer. My first thought is, *Is this cancer? Has it spread?* ... and then my logical brain jumps in and says no, this is not cancer ... so in some ways, everything feels like cancer, yet nothing feels like cancer.

I did get some reassuring news from my breast surgeon. They were meticulous about removal of breast tissue – so where other surgeons may leave a little more, she scrapes the skin thin to remove all the breast tissue – sometimes this causes skin death. I have a small patch that didn't make it, which then becomes the plastic surgeon's job to fix. I'm OK with that. If a 'local recurrence' were to happen, it could be on the skin itself or on the chest wall. Both are very rare – they don't even screen for the chest wall recurrence. My next visit with my breast surgeon is in 6-months (yay).

My oncologist also made me feel better about my other aches and pains. My worries about spread being so unlikely (but hey – so is bilateral breast cancer) ... but still. I was informed that there is a 1-3% chance of improved survival with ovarian suppression and Aromatase Inhibitors (AIs) over Tamoxifen in pre-menopausal women (note that it is an increase of 1-3% not an improvement of 1-3%. This means that if survival is 70% then the increase is (.7*.1 to .7*.3) or 70.7-72.1% (I think I did that correctly). This is causing the clinical oncology world to question which treatment option to be recommending. I'm going to start off with the Tamoxifen and see how things go. Both Tamoxifen and AIs have side effects, and I don't like the AI side effect of increased risk of osteoporosis – where Tamoxifen helps your bones grow stronger. We shall see how it all goes. I've been told I can wait a little longer before starting Tamoxifen (a couple more weeks) to better recover from the surgery, so I have some time to further ponder. Today, I went on the same bike ride as yesterday, on my Bike Friday – which is faster than the trike. The distance was almost 6km, and it took 23 minutes. The tension on my arms was a little more than I'd like, so I will give the Bike Friday a rest for a few days (or until next week). My knees feel better, but still hurt a bit when I bike. If you had told me at this time last year that I'd be struggling to ride 6km I'd have laughed at you. But, alas, I am taking it one step (or pedal stroke) at a time.

Breast that are not breasts[2]

———

January 27, 2015

I have breasts that are not breasts. They look like breasts. They feel like breasts. But are they really breasts?

When I look down, my chest appears normal. But my nipples no longer have sensation or reaction. My chest does not recognize or feel its own boundaries.

Imagine what your face feels like after going to the dentist for a filling. You know your face is still there, but it does not have feeling. After breast cancer and surgeries, I look down and see that my breasts are there. I touch them with my hands. I feel that they are warm. But they are numb—just like after the dentist. Only, my body will never regrow nerves there. I will never have feeling in my chest again.

I first noticed the lack of sensation when I was carrying a box upstairs. The box was light, but bulky. When I held it, I had no sense of where my body ended. I could not tell how much pressure I was using with my arms, because I could not sense the pressure on my chest.

I was reminded of it again when I did a chair massage at the cancer centre. When I climbed into the chair and leaned forward, I had to visually check to see if I was positioned correctly. I did not have the sensory cue to tell me that I was leaning against something.

It is odd not having feeling in my chest. For many breast cancer patients, our surgeons never mentioned this, and I have no recollection of my surgeon mentioning it. I had read about it, so I thought I was prepared, but really, I was not. While not having sensation in my chest means that I cannot feel the horrible wounds as they heal, it is still disconcerting. It is not limited to being unable to feel silicone or saline implants. Having had a flap reconstruction that took part of my stomach tissue to recreate my breasts, my breasts are truly a part of my body, my blood flows through them, they are warm, and yet, they do not have feeling.

The impact of not having feeling is starting to settle in. Eight weeks after surgery, I am finally allowed to lie on my stomach. The first time I try it, I feel very scared. Am I causing harm? Is there something underneath, which, unknowingly to me, might poke into me? Am I tearing open my wound? How do I possibly get comfortable when I cannot feel?

When I ask about what a breast self-exam looks like with flap-reconstructed breasts, both my breast surgeon and my oncologist tell me, "They are not breasts."

I have breasts that are not breasts.

[2] This story was published in *Shivering in a paper gown: Breast cancer and its aftermath: An Anthology*. Eds. Calari Campbell, Pomeranz, Ziba, 2015.

When do I get to say, 'I had breast cancer?'

February 2, 2015

I did it. I opened the package, examined the small pill, and then swallowed it. For the next 10 years I'll be taking a pill to reduce my body's production of estrogen, which is what was feeding my cancer. Tamoxifen is used to significantly decrease the likelihood of recurrence – mostly used in pre-menopausal women who had hormone positive cancer. After menopause, the drug group of choice are known as Aromatase inhibitors (AIs). It is expected that after a couple of years on Tamoxifen, I'll be switched over to AIs as they may be more effective. It is a bit of a game of side effects – not sure which is better or worse.

I was struggling with the idea of Tamoxifen until just the other day. My mother-in-law has tried to convince me for months that Tamoxifen isn't evil, it is not bad, it is nothing like chemotherapy or surgery – rather just something you do. It is something that works for you, to help keep the cancer from returning. But then she said something that worked for me – it works on your body in mostly the same way hormonal birth control does. I had no trouble taking hormonal birth control, so why should I have difficulty with tamoxifen? For me, that worked. It is interesting the things that stick and the things that don't. I know for many women, Tamoxifen has had negative side effects, but so have AIs, and cancer really sucks too. For some, maybe it is just the idea that it is a pill a day (somewhat larger than birth control pills). The fact that blocks estrogen in a way that is not dissimilar to the way birth control blocks ovulation works for me. I can do this.

The information pamphlet explains that the medication is used to treat breast cancer. I don't have breast cancer anymore! When do I get to start staying *that I **had** breast cancer rather than I **have** breast cancer?* In my mind, that date was December 17, 2014 – the day that I had a double mastectomy and the last of my three tumours was removed along with any other breast tissue. The pathology confirmed that all my margins were clear – meaning that there was enough healthy tissue surrounding the cancerous tissue to indicate that they got it all.

I don't **have** breast cancer, I **had** it.

That being said, I'm still undergoing treatment as a result of breast cancer. My cancer surgery is done. I've graduated to 6-month checkups with my breast surgeon. My chemotherapy is done. However, my reconstruction is not yet finished. I still have a couple of gaping wounds that will require another surgery to clean up. I'm weak from the chemotherapy and the surgery. I've lost a lot of my muscle mass. I'm working on getting it all back, but recovery is anything but over. Although I'm done with the active treatment **for** cancer, I'm not done with the treatment **because of** cancer.

When do I get to say I had breast cancer?

Afterward

As of 17 December 2021, I have been cancer free for seven years. For some reason, that feels like a significant milestone in my cancer journey. I hope to one day move onto the next part of my story – the year after treatment, which I found to be more difficult than the year of treatment, but I also had a lot of breakthroughs with my mental health that are worth sharing. If you want to read a detailed account of my story, the original blog remains at https://bcbecky.com[1].

I have since left California and moved back to Canada, to a small town in Nova Scotia. My California oncologist has retired. My Nova Scotia oncologist has graduated me to yearly checkups. I'm still taking tamoxifen, but that is a story for another time.

For now, I enjoy my days walking on the beach, hiking, and teaching online. My family has grown to include a small dog, who we named Cali for California. She is cuteness personified.

---

1. https://bcbecky.com/

Don't miss out!

Visit the website below and you can sign up to receive emails whenever Rebecca J Hogue publishes a new book. There's no charge and no obligation.

https://books2read.com/r/B-A-IZAW-REHVC

BOOKS 2 READ

Connecting independent readers to independent writers.

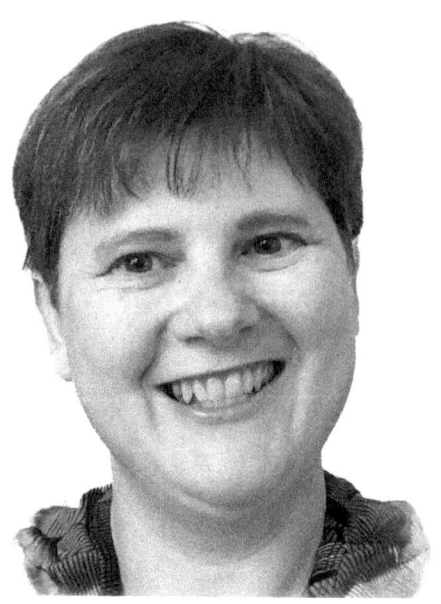

About the Author

Rebecca J. Hogue began blogging when she and her husband took 16 months off and rode their bikes and travelled around the world without airplanes. When she was diagnosed with breast cancer at 43, she started blogging about her lived experience. Professionally she is an author and an instructional designer. Rebecca and her husband now live in Nova Scotia Canada.

Read more at https://rebeccahogue.com/memoir/.